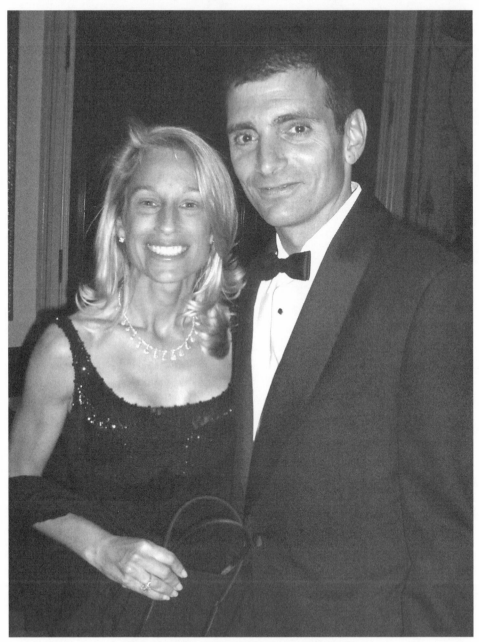

Mark & Cathy - Three years after diagnosis

WHEN YOUR WIFE HAS
BREAST CANCER

A STORY OF LOVE, COURAGE,
AND SURVIVAL

MARK S.WEISS

ibooks
new york
www.ibooks.net

DISTRIBUTED BY PUBLISHERS GROUP WEST

A Publication of ibooks, inc.

Distributed by:
Publishers Group West
1700 Fourth Street, Berkeley, CA 94710

ibooks, inc.
24 West 25th Street
New York, NY 10010

Cover photo by Leslie Erlich

ISBN 1-59687-313-2
First ibooks, inc. printing February 2006
10 9 8 7 6 5 4 3

Printed in the U.S.A.

Table of Contents

DEDICATION

To Doctor Chau Dang, Cathy's oncologist, who treated Cathy with brilliance and tenderness.

To Jeannette and Eugene Weiss, my parents, who but for themselves were so very alone fighting my mom's breast cancer in 1969.

To my precious boys Brandon, Ryan and their older brother Or who made it impossible for us not to endure and boldly face all challenges.

To Cathy Weiss, my treasured wife, who redefined grace, courage and selflessness and taught me to be a better man.

Byron Preiss
1953-2005

The man who believed in this book and the importance of its message.
I am forever grateful.

Preface

By

Linda Fairstein

After I first learned the news that my friend Cathy Weiss had been diagnosed with breast cancer, I found myself constantly studying the photograph of Cathy and Mark that hung on a bulletin board over my writing desk. It had been taken at a charity benefit earlier in the year, and it captured much of the vitality and attractiveness of this wonderful young couple who seemed to have it all.

They are smart and warm young adults, loving parents of two adorable sons, with an army of loyal friends. Mark's business successes allowed them to involve themselves with great energy and generosity in a number of important causes. Cathy deserved the happiness and good health that always seemed to radiate from her. I knew she had been a sexual assault survivor and sort of figured that she'd suffered enough trauma and had more than given back with her work. She deserved every good thing that came her way, and the devastating news delivered by the physicians just didn't fit with the smiling faces that beamed out at me from the photograph.

The news got worse. First was the diagnosis of the malignancy, followed by word that a complete mastectomy would be required. After that, the research revealed a genetic predisposition to this type of cancer, which suggested the removal of both breasts.

As usual, family and friends rallied around Cathy, while she, of course, looked to her beloved Mark to get her through the ordeal of the months that followed.

It didn't take Mark very long to learn that there was no blueprint to guide them through the battle of their lives. As a devoted husband and a strong business professional, Mark convinced Cathy to plan a goal - to make a resolve that they would fight this cancer as a team, with every emotional resource available - in order to reach that goal of disease-free survival.

In this brilliantly candid book, Mark Weiss explores with us his challenges and distress, his insecurities and his anger, his determination and his overarching desire to help make Cathy well.

A lot has been written to give guidance to the women—over 200,000 of them every year in the United States—who are diagnosed with this disease. And although seventy-five percent of the 2.8 million women who are living with breast cancer in this country now are married, very little in the literature reflects the impact of the diagnosis and treatment on their husbands.

We learn from Mark about his natural instinct to want to protect his wife and sons, to add to his roles of husband, father and provider the jobs of caregiver and 'mother' to his kids as well. His object was to support Cathy in the fight of her life, for her life—and do that while overseeing all the necessary financial adjustments and child care arrangements, participating in medical decisions that might profoundly alter their relationship, and finding some kind of outlet for his own denial, his own frustration, his own vulnerabilities.

Cathy has described Mark's approach to her illness as creating a methodical intensity that amazed her. As she struggled through surgery, the postoperative pain issues, reconstructive surgery, and chemotherapy with the very little strength she had left she watched Mark try to wrestle with the uncontrollable-holding himself to impossible standards and expectations that she feared would weaken him to the point of breaking.

The story that Mark Weiss tells in this book is incredibly honest and informative, and is a primer for anyone in a relationship whose partner is diagnosed with a life-threatening illness. It is a love story, and a tale of triumph over adversity, full of practical advice reinforced by the real-life lessons Mark learned during Cathy's crisis and their joint recovery to good health.

DECEMBER 12, 2002, OUR RAINY DAY

I was in my midtown Manhattan office, on the phone and with two calls on hold. Business was really good, and I was completely energized by the pressure and excitement of finishing several intricate projects by year's end. My cell phone rang in the breast pocket of my suit jacket; caller ID told me it was Cathy, calling from her cell. She never called me in the morning. After thirteen years of marriage, our life had certain rhythms, and this was outside of that rhythm. I immediately felt that it wouldn't be good news.

"Mark, I don't know how to tell you this, so I'll just tell you… I have a malignant tumor on my breast." There was an eerie calmness to her voice, as if she was talking about someone else.

"Where are you?" I asked her.

"Barbara Edelstein's office."

"Where is that?"

"1086 Park Avenue, on 87th Street."

"I'll be right there. We'll take care of this." I put down the phone and immediately pictured my wife, as she looked that morning: a beautiful, confident woman, and mother of our two young boys—Brandon, 8, and Ryan, 3. She was so strong, so vibrant, and never sick.

Memories began to flood my mind. I remembered Cathy as a stunning young California girl who was new to New York and answered my ad for a roommate fifteen years earlier-how my heart stopped when I first saw her, and how we grew from strangers to lovers, then to husband and wife, and finally to best friends. Cathy spent all of her energy caring for and about others. It hit me that she was about to go through a battle for her own life, and that I would need to be with her every step of the way. I raced out of the office without even collecting my things.

A few minutes later, I arrived at the doctor's office, out of breath, and met Cathy. Sitting with our hands locked, we were in simultaneous states of shock and denial as I asked Dr. Edelstein, the diagnosing radiologist, "How can you tell this is malignant from a mammogram without a biopsy?" I think she was initially surprised that someone would challenge or question her, but then she confidently explained that, based on all of her years of experience, I should not hold out hope that this was anything but a malignancy. The tumor was palpable, spiculated and presented classically, almost out of a textbook. I later learned that a spiculated tumor is one with jagged or star-shaped edges-characteristics that are consistent with a malignancy. If a tumor has round or smooth edges, there is a great chance of it being benign.

"Mark, you deal with this right away," the doctor urged. "See a surgeon as soon as possible as delaying could be disastrous."

While Cathy was changing in the next room, I asked Dr. Edelstein if my wife would survive. I could see in her face that she was taken aback by the frankness of my question and the immediate grasp I had of the gravity of the situation we were facing. In hindsight, I suppose she is accustomed to dispensing harsh or blunt advice to shell-shocked patients. I was shell shocked too, but I still had questions! Her surprise at my reaction notwithstanding, her answer was short and to the point: "Yes, she'll survive, but she is in for a miserable year." As I walked out of her office, she added, "Cathy is both lucky and smart that she has had annual mammograms since she was thirty."

Most women don't have mammograms until they are forty years old because that seems to be the recommendation of the insurance companies. When Cathy turned thirty, the gynecologist she was seeing, Dr. Sanford Sullum, strongly encouraged her to start getting mammograms because he wasn't convinced by the available statistical data that it wasn't necessary.

I related well to Dr. Edelstein's confidence; in my business I, too, try to be as straightforward and unambiguous as possible when dispensing advice in my profession, commercial real estate brokerage in New York City. There are times that I know, based on experience, how events will likely unfold for a client on a particular deal. At these times, clear and sometimes blunt communication is appropriate. If a diagnosing radiologist is vague or unclear, it could play into a patient's natural defense mechanism of denial and cause them to delay potentially life-saving treatment. Barbara Edelstein did her job successfully because we left her office with the knowledge that this was a potentially lethal situation, and that any denial or delay could cost Cathy her life.

The chances of this not going to the top of our priority lists were zero. While I had tried to show no fear for Cathy—and perhaps for myself—Dr. Edelstein had scared the hell out of me. I realized that the informational advantage she had over us in an area where we desperately needed information was gargantuan. We later learned that although Dr. Edelstein's peers regard her as an excellent radiologist and diagnostician, radiologists in general aren't trained to be especially compassionate or reassuring, but to be meticulous diagnosticians and effective communicators. She was both.

Cathy was grateful that I was there to process the gravity of the news we were given that morning. Like many other patients, she froze after the initial diagnosis and didn't absorb the explanation and advice that followed. In fact, she may not have even heard it since her world, our world, was changing in a horrifying way.

We walked the ten blocks to our home on 79th Street as if we were drugged. It was an unseasonably mild December morning and we kept our coats open. But we were fighting panic, so we barely noticed that it was a beautiful day as we struggled to be strong for each other. When we got to our apartment, I pulled out a spiral notebook and started to draft a plan. Cathy asked me what I was doing, and I explained that we needed to figure this thing out so that we could use our time intelligently. I said, "Cathy, we have to draft a plan with a goal and a starting point." This is how I always solved problems, but I wasn't sure if this disease was something I could solve and that terrified me.

Any good plan starts with a goal, and we started with just that. On page one of my notebook, I wrote *Our Goal: To Survive*. Cathy and I resolved to do whatever was necessary to ensure survival, or at least enhance the chances of it to whatever degree we could. Only later, as we learned more about cancer did we restate our goal to Disease-Free Survival. I remember saying to Cathy while we were sitting at our dining room table less than an hour after her diagnosis, "If this goes against us and I find myself holding your hand in a hospital room while you are dying, we're not going to be talking about what we should have done more aggressively or decisively to beat this thing. We've got to agree to fight this cancer with everything we have." Cathy immediately agreed and cried softly. I choked back tears for a minute or so, as I watched the enormity of Cathy's visit with Barbara Edelstein take hold. We then got to work drafting our plan.

Introduction

We knew that we needed a biopsy and would need to see a breast surgeon as soon as possible. We also knew that Christmas was coming up in two weeks and that most doctors would be going away on vacation. Getting access to surgeons right before Christmas, and on relatively short notice, required focus, a bit of persuasiveness, resourcefulness, connections and luck.

Cathy is remarkable in that she does so much and does it all so well. In addition to starting and running her own executive recruiting business, plus being involved in every aspect of our children's lives and educations, Cathy is a volunteer at Mount Sinai Hospital where she serves as a New York State licensed crisis counselor assisting survivors of sexual assault and domestic violence for an organization called SAVI (Sexual Assault and Violence Intervention program). She is also on SAVI's Board of Directors and an avid fundraiser for this important organization. This position, coupled with her position on the Auxiliary Board of Mount Sinai Hospital, allowed her access to several Board members of the hospital, where SAVI is based.

Cathy's friend and fellow SAVI board member, Nancy Aronson, helped us secure an appointment with a surgeon from Mount Sinai for the next day. Through another close friend and SAVI Board member, Katie Horowitz, Cathy was introduced to Evelyn Lauder, the principal benefactor of The Breast Center at Memorial Sloan Kettering Cancer Center (MSKCC). The Breast Center is a separate part of MSKCC, housed in a building four blocks from the main hospital, and its entire staff is dedicated exclusively to the treatment and needs of women facing breast cancer. Mrs. Lauder not only got us access, but also made some very helpful recommendations relative to choosing a surgeon. Meanwhile, the CEO of my firm, Barry Gosin, has represented MSKCC on several complicated and successful real estate acquisitions, and he used his contacts there to make certain that we were being treated as if we were friends of MSKCC.

Many people, myself included, are reticent about asking people for favors or for using connections for anything other than arranging a favor for someone else. But when you are confronted with cancer in your family, you pull out all the stops and use whatever connections you have to get access to the right medical care. There is no reason to save the favor or contact; a diagnosis of cancer has more urgency and impact than pretty much all of life's other problems.

Before we left Barbara Edelstein's office, she had recommended a very well respected breast surgeon at New York Hospital. We called for an appointment and were pleased to find out that he had a cancellation for the following Tuesday. We were moving quickly and with a focused sense of intensity because we wanted to define Cathy's surgical future before Christmas. We both felt that every day we delayed increased the probability of a spread of this pernicious disease and would diminish our chances of securing our goal—*disease-free survival.* Fortunately, breast surgeons are generally accustomed to promptly seeing people who call them with a recent diagnosis of breast cancer.

We soon discovered that interviewing surgeons was a relatively expensive proposition because, while we had insurance, all were "out of network," and we had to first pay each doctor and hope to get reimbursed. There wasn't even enough time to check with our insurance company to see what consultations they would or wouldn't reimburse. My attitude was to pay each doctor on the spot and argue later—with our insurance company, if necessary. I was focused on understanding Cathy's cancer, and wasn't going to let our insurance company dictate how we attacked it. My instincts told me that our insurance company would have a different agenda than the Weiss'. We felt like we were drowning and weren't about to negotiate the price of lifejackets. We decided to use our medical consultations as a means to choose a surgeon and to learn as much as possible about breast cancer. As long as you are not in a state of total panic, you can learn a tremendous amount from a one-hour interview with a surgeon, provided the surgeon is a good communicator.

Without discussing it with Cathy, I also immediately started to focus on the financial consequences of Cathy's cancer. Instinctively, I knew that financial pressure could cause us to make emotional decisions that could be catastrophic. I needed to accept that a portion of the money I had saved to get us through any slow business periods might be spent on this crisis. We had always lived conservatively relative to income and saved money for a rainy day. *December 12 was our rainy day.* For me, segregating money for Cathy's treatment and its aftermath was an important part of the acceptance that my wife had cancer.

I remembered seeing a news program some years ago about a couple who went bankrupt paying for "experimental treatments" intended to save the wife's life. The story centered on a couple in Massachusetts, where the wife was fighting a losing battle with breast cancer. At the time, bone marrow transplants were regarded as promising but experimental. They remortgaged their home and maxed out their credit cards with cash advances to pay for this treatment as a final hope for saving her life. They simultaneously battled cancer and their insurance company, which steadfastly refused to acknowledge the promise of this type of therapy because they didn't want to set a precedent of paying for it. In the end, she died, leaving a heartbroken husband and two grieving children in both emotional and financial ruin.

With this irrational fear, I called my bank to expand my home equity line of credit in the event that I would need cash quickly. Before December 12, I really liked having little to no debt in my life; the lack of financial pressure allowed me to make better business choices and advocate for clients in a totally objective manner because I never felt any fee-driven pressure. But after Cathy's diagnosis, I wanted to concentrate on getting her healthy, and not on how to pay for it.

Our plan was coming together. We had a defined goal, mapped out the major steps toward achieving that goal, and had a basic idea how to pay for it, save for the high hopes I had that our insurance company would be cooperative.

CHAPTER 2

CHOOSING A SURGEON

The next morning—Thursday, December 13—we had our first appointment with a very well regarded surgeon from Mount Sinai Hospital. I had arranged to meet Cathy at the surgeon's office, which wasn't far from our apartment. As I was walking there, my friend Jerry Larkin called me on my cell phone just to say hello. He was unaware of Cathy's recent diagnosis. I remember telling him what was going on, that we were about to find out how Cathy's tumor would be treated, and how we were hopeful that a lumpectomy and a little radiation would solve our problem. Jerry told me that he would pray for us. He immediately grasped the gravity of what we were about to face.

We arrived at the appointment on time and gave the receptionist Cathy's mammogram films, and then waited unproductively for about three quarters of an hour until the surgeon could see us. Although the surgeon was well respected in medical circles, we didn't connect with her on any level; the chemistry between us just wasn't right. Our appointment started in a lighthearted way, with the surgeon initiating a few minutes of small talk. I remember thinking that if she were going to deliver bad news, she wouldn't have started with "Upper East Side chit chat." The discussion ranged from apartments to children and schools. She then put the mammogram films on a light box that was mounted on the wall next to her desk. My heart started to race in nervous anticipation as I realized by the way she started to study the films that she hadn't looked at them before this moment. Her pleasant, even lighthearted demeanor changed quite suddenly, which terrified both Cathy and me; we knew she had seen something that we weren't going to like.

After explaining to us how a breast worked, the surgeon showed us on the films that, based on the location of the obviously malignant tumor; breast conservation surgery was not realistic. I looked at Cathy and saw that she didn't process this last statement so I asked the surgeon to repeat it for both of us. She then slowly explained that based on the location of the tumor, the size of Cathy's breast and the need for cutting a clear margin around a tumor meant that a lumpectomy would not be sufficient. Cathy would have a mastectomy; she would lose her right breast. Hearing this made Cathy's cancer horrifyingly real.

We hugged and looked at each other with helpless, tear-filled eyes as we sat across the desk from a surgeon we had met only fifteen minutes earlier. She explained things well, but again I was at a tremendous informational disadvantage because I understood very little about breasts and even less about cancer. I didn't even completely understand what a mastectomy was from a surgical point-of-view.

I think most men believe that a mastectomy is a breast amputation. It is not! Surgeons don't cut off a woman's breast; at least, they don't do it that way now. Breast tissue lies under the skin and above the pectoralis muscle in a woman's chest. It is made up of lobules, glands, connective tissue, ducts and a duct opening, or nipple. A layer of fat surrounds this tissue, which is intertwined with the pectoralis muscle. In a mastectomy, the surgeon cuts open the skin, removes the nipple and carefully cuts out the surrounding fat and breast tissue. A skilled surgeon can remove most, but not all, of the breast tissue. What remains afterward is a fair amount of skin and a pocket in a woman's chest that previously held breast tissue and the surrounding fat. The surplus skin and the pocket make breast reconstruction possible. Since many women choose to have reconstruction immediately after mastectomies, breast surgeons and reconstructive plastic surgeons often work in teams. The reconstructive surgeon starts working as the breast surgeon is finishing. Therefore, we needed to meet a reconstructive surgeon and learn how they would reconstruct Cathy's right breast and how it would be matched to the left one.

That afternoon, the breast surgeon from Mount Sinai was able to get us an immediate appointment with a reconstructive plastic surgeon with whom she frequently worked. He had a calming way about him and was methodical in how he explained the process of breast reconstruction and the options available to us. He immediately assessed that Cathy was too thin to have TRAM Flap reconstruction and would have her breast reconstructed using a tissue expander. TRAM Flap reconstruction is reconstructive surgery in which a woman's abdominal muscle is pulled up (inside the body, of course) to create a breast mound. Tissue expanders are temporary implants that are inserted during the mastectomy under the pectoralis and seriates muscles, then get expanded every two weeks or so by injecting saline through a valve. Later, after chemotherapy ended (if chemo was necessary), another surgery would replace the expanders with permanent implants filled with either saline or silicone.

We also learned at this appointment that the nipples would be constructed at a later surgery, since no mastectomy can conserve the nipple. Simply pinching and stitching the skin together would make the nipples, while the areolae would be created from a skin graft taken from Cathy's tummy, groin or buttocks. In addition to these surgeries, Cathy's new nipples and areola would later be tattooed to complete the look of her newly constructed breasts.

After just a few short hours, we were on information overload. I knew then that I needed to learn more about this so that I could help make intelligent decisions that were not clouded by confusion and emotion.

At that point my emotions were telling me that we should just let this doctor from Mount Sinai operate on Cathy, as she seemed competent, was well regarded and was available to operate the very next week. I shared these thoughts with Cathy as we left her office, but to her great credit, she insisted on following the plan that we had just drafted the day before: *"Interview surgeons, learn as much as possible, then choose the best possible team."* Choosing a team meant considering more than just one surgeon, and doing so with a basis of knowledge and preparation!

I'm glad Cathy had the presence of mind to force us to adhere to the plan rather than be guided by the easy emotional answer, which was to treat cancer care as a commodity and *"just get rid of it."* In hindsight, that would have been a mistake, as we later learned that surgery and oncology are not fungible. There are dramatic qualitative differences in both, which is demonstrated by examining the survival rates of different cancer hospitals. The short exchange Cathy and I had on choosing a team set the tone for all of our decision making relative to medical choices. We would collaborate on all decisions, and Cathy would welcome and value my input, but all final decisions would be hers. I assessed that my role would be to ferret out all important facts and issues, then present them to Cathy in a manner that would allow for the best possible decisions. I knew at that point that while I would have significant input, Cathy would choose a surgeon who felt right to her on both a rational and emotional level.

The next day, Friday, was biopsy day. The biopsy was both scary and painful; the radiologist, after making sure that I paid her upfront, held out no hope that this was anything but a malignant tumor. She radiated no personal warmth, nor did her demeanor inspire any confidence. Getting paid up front must be common practice for radiologists and mammographers because once a tumor is found; it is improbable that the patient will ever come back to that radiologist and, who might feel awkward asking for $750 from a woman who just found out that she has a malignancy. While

Choosing a Surgeon

Cathy's tumor appeared to be malignant from the mammogram pictures, the biopsy and its subsequent report would reveal the type of cancer cells and how they would likely progress, including whether they were well or poorly differentiated, and whether or not they were infiltrating. The pathology report, which uses information from the tissue taken during the biopsy, tells the oncologist the likely effect certain types of chemotherapy drugs might have later on. A more complete report, derived from the breast tissue taken during surgery, comes later.

Cathy's biopsy was sent to Mount Sinai Hospital, where it was set in paraffin wax, thin-sliced, stained and then studied under a microscope. It was painstakingly compared to the mammogram films where the microscopic tumor cells and calcifications were first matched against each other, evaluated, defined and finally dictated into Cathy's pathology report—literally a report card on her cancer. We had no idea then, but having Dr. Ira Bleiweiss do the pathology report was a blessing because he is truly a doctor's detective. In no way is a pathology report purely objective. There is much subjectivity in evaluating the subtle nuances of a small sample of breast tissue.

There are actually four different ways to biopsy a lump on a woman's breast: fine needle, large needle, excisional and incisional. Cathy had her biopsy with a large needle and it hurt like hell. I sat outside the room with her dearest friend Caryl, while a doctor and two nurses attended to Cathy. As she cried out in pain, Caryl and I looked at each other helplessly, horrified that we couldn't even be there to hold her hand. I had asked to be in the room, but the radiologist was adamant that she didn't want me there. One of the attending nurses later explained their concern was that a non-medically trained person might get squeamish and actually faint in the room, which would impair their ability to focus on the important task.

For Cathy's biopsy, the radiologist used an ultrasound scanner to guide the large needle into the tumor. Once located, and provided it wasn't on the surface, the tumor was aspirated with the needle. This aspiration extracted the cancer cells that would tell us what type of cancer we were facing. If Cathy's biopsy had any prospect of a result other than being a "malignant tumor," perhaps it wouldn't have been as physically and emotionally painful for her.

That afternoon, we confirmed two more surgical appointments for the following week. The first appointment would be on Monday with the surgeon from New York Hospital who was referred to us by Barbara Edelstein. The next appointment would be on Tuesday with Dr. Alexandra Heerdt of Memorial Sloan Kettering Cancer Center. It was a cloudy, cold Friday afternoon and I was drained, but I couldn't show any strain because our young children would soon be home from school and would have picked up on it.

Friday nights in our home are typically spent together as a family. In fact, on most Friday evenings we light candles to welcome the Sabbath, even though we don't observe it beyond Friday night dinner. Cathy and I almost never go out on a Friday evening, as we are both generally exhausted from a full week of pretty much constant activity. One of our rituals during dinner is that we go around the table and talk about our "highs" and "lows" of the week. We initially started doing this as a way to encourage the boys to express themselves and to hear about whatever mattered to them. Since we all reported on our "highs" and "lows," Cathy and I had to be especially creative in making up a 'low', because this week's was a real showstopper! I simply had to go about Friday evening as usual and knew that I had the entire weekend, starting after the boys went to sleep, to learn as much as possible about breast cancer, surgery and reconstruction. Seeing as I would have time later to educate myself about chemotherapy, focusing my learning on surgery was the pressing issue.

That night I had only the Internet as a source of information, which was unfortunate because the information on the Internet is completely fragmented. Much of it is also horribly written, being either too general or too specific. Compounding matters was that pharmaceutical companies advocating their products posted much of the information as a thinly veiled exercise in selling their "incredibly effective" drugs.

We went into the weekend reasonably certain that there was no genetic predisposition toward cancer in Cathy's family. Barbara Edelstein and Cathy's gynecologist before her, Dr. Jean Chin, had asked Cathy about a family history for breast cancer and appeared satisfied with her answer that Cathy's maternal aunt, Bryna, had died two years earlier from a form of breast cancer called inflammatory breast disease. Cathy was very close to her aunt, and watching her die such a difficult death contributed to Cathy's general state of terror regarding her own diagnosis. The plastic surgeon and the radiologist who biopsied Cathy's breast also asked her about family history, and both received the same answer. In fact, all the doctors we saw asked the same question and were given Cathy's usual answer about Aunt Bryna, which appeared to satisfy them because they went on to other questions.

The answer, however, was given without much deep thought, which is pretty much how the question was asked. Neither of us had focused on the family history part of cancer because we were new to this and didn't yet understand the importance of the BRCA-1 or BRCA-2 genes. The presence of these genes is a strong indicator as to whether a woman is likely to develop breast and/or ovarian cancer in her lifetime. In thinking back to the doctors' questions regarding family history, it reminded me of being queried by an airport security guard—pre-9/11—if anyone had given me an explosive device or any other package with unknown contents and had asked me to take it on the plane. The question was asked in a perfunctory way, and the answer was invariably disregarded.

Looking back, I now believe that doctors should present the family history question in this manner: "The progression of your cancer, its treatment surgically and beyond, will be largely governed by genetic markers. Genetic testing takes time, and since time is of the essence right now, we really need to investigate whether there has been either breast or ovarian cancer in your family. Focus on your father and mother's family and go back a few generations, if possible. If need be, use my phone to call your parents, even if you are not on speaking terms with them. Call them, and then fill out this template of a family tree. The information you provide here can help you avoid the unnecessary risk of a second surgery and metastasis." Or perhaps, while sitting in a doctor's reception area after filling out insurance forms (which is largely irrelevant, since many of the doctors we saw don't take payment from the insurance companies), they should simply have a family tree template and ask you to fill it out, writing "BC" next to anyone who has or has had breast cancer or "PD" next to any woman who suffered a premature death of unknown cause. This exercise would be productive for doctor and patient, and would make the agonizing wait at the doctor's office highly productive.

Doctors sometimes forget to enlist and empower their patients into the diagnosis and treatment of illness and disease. Enlisting the patient could put a medical investigation on the right path sooner by providing the doctor with valuable information.

Each doctor did ask Cathy when she had her first child, as well as when she first had her period. It wasn't until much later that we learned that the greater the time period between menstruation and pregnancy correlated to a greater propensity for a woman developing breast cancer. During the first thirty-six hours after diagnosis, there was no shortage of information being thrust at us.

We had already called our families to let them know what we were up against. My parents are married and live in Florida. My in-laws live in Los Angeles where Cathy grew up. My mother-in-law Phyllis is typically a very emotional person, but was actually calm and productive—at least for the first forty-eight hours after being told. She took it upon herself to do histories of both her family and her ex-husband Jason's. Through some extensive investigating, which included phone calls to long lost dysfunctional former relatives she came up with nine breast cancer deaths on Jason's side of the family. Ironically, my father-in-law, a litigator by training, wasn't able to provide us with this insight. At the time, I was a little disappointed with Jason; I felt he should have been resourceful enough to provide us with this type of insight into his family. He must have frozen when he heard from three thousand miles away that his only daughter was stricken with a potentially fatal disease. Phyllis, however, used this information as a springboard for productive action despite her sense of terror over having a daughter with cancer after just losing her sister to the disease.

That night, using the information that Phyllis had pooled together, I created Cathy's family tree in our cancer notebook. All breast, chest or ovarian cancers were colored green. By the time we were finished, there was a lot of green. It was unambiguous to us—Cathy had a genetic predisposition toward breast cancer, as most of the cancers were on her father's side of the family. These were people who lived and died in Massachusetts, which is where both Phyllis and Jason met. Jason had never been close to his family and had very little contact with them since he moved to California with Phyllis some forty years earlier, shortly after he finished law school. Cathy never knew many of these people and certainly didn't associate them as "family," which is why she never correctly answered any of her doctors' queries regarding family history.

We realized that Cathy was a walking time bomb because she had no idea that she was genetically predetermined to develop breast cancer.

Emotionally, we think of family as people we know and love, but for the purposes of investigating a family history for cancer, love and Thanksgiving dinners mean nothing. DNA is the only meaningful marker. While this may seem perfectly obvious, it isn't immediately apparent to a woman waiting in her doctor's office after being examined for a lump in her breast. At this point, her mind is racing and she's not thinking clearly enough to consider *all* blood relatives—not just the ones she knows and loves—as family unless she is specifically instructed to do so.

That evening, I got a sneak preview of my sleeping patterns for the next year or so. I was surprised that I fell asleep easily and that it was a black, dreamless sleep. Unfortunately, I woke up completely wired only five hours later. As soon as my eyes opened, I knew that I was up for the day. After waiting for the rest of New York City to wake up that Saturday morning, I went to Barnes & Noble because I was disgusted with all the unfiltered and unformatted crap that I found on the Internet. I wanted basic facts and knowledge about breast cancer, surgery, reconstruction and chemotherapy. I needed to understand how a woman's breast worked, and what happened to it when it was attacked by cancer. This understanding would afford me the ability to be clearheaded, listen to surgeons more effectively and help Cathy make intelligent decisions regarding treatment going forward.

Initially, I was impressed by the amount of reading material that I found on this topic. I wanted two types of books. First and foremost, a book that was replete with up-to-date medical information on breast cancer and a very comprehensive glossary. I would use the glossary to help me translate the pathology report and familiarize myself with the phrases and words that I had heard over the past two days. Words like ductal, lobular, acini, fibroadenomas, in-situ, infiltrating, invasive, neoplasm, tram flap, tissue expanders, chemotherapy, radiation, local and distant metastases were new to me. I needed to understand them and know what they meant because it would help me process the barrage of new information we were receiving. I also was hoping to find a short, easy-to-read basic playbook for husbands supporting a wife through these difficult times. The former was easy to find. The latter was not.

Up until this point, all of the learning was from our interactions with physicians who presented their points-of-view and exposed us to what they wanted us to know, and when they wanted us to know it. I realized that receiving information from doctors only is sub-optimal. It is illogical to think that a physician could have the same values that we have or the same outlook on life. Their unique values as human beings invariably leads them to slant any advice they give to a patient to reflect their outlook on life. And most physicians will not say things like, "I only handle fifteen cases like this a year, and if it were my wife who was ill, I'd go to someone who sees fifteen cases like this a month."

Being armed with good, solid information before interviewing physicians is both smart and productive, which is why I engaged in the process of finding a surgeon while giving myself a crash course in breast cancer—its consequences and how it might be treated. The vexing part of this "education" was the constant awareness that the clock was ticking against us. I was also acutely aware that I would need an intensity of focus during this crash course so that I could separate emotion from reason and help Cathy make smart choices.

In that regard, I didn't broadcast our predicament to many people because I was fearful that we would be bombarded with well-meaning suggestions, that were intended to help us, but could actually delay, or worse, sidetrack our education. I was really concerned that friends, family or coworkers would start dispensing medical advice or suggesting dietary changes. One colleague at work who had heard early on about our medical challenges approached me real sweetly with obvious concern in her eyes, even though I didn't know her very well. She went on to tell me that her older sister had breast cancer, then started to suggest some sort of alternative medicine like eating tofu mixed with broccoli or something equally inane, given where I was at that point in the cancer process. I nicely stated that while I knew she was trying to be helpful, my wife was facing a medical crisis and we were investigating treatment alternatives through professional channels in an organized and methodical way.

Some people, however well meaning, offer offhand suggestions, perhaps to make themselves feel better. More important, while other people say things to us like "I am so impressed with the way you are handling this. You are both in my prayers." I learned quickly that less is more when it comes to expressions of support.

After searching the women's health section in Barnes & Noble, I bought five books. The two that I most strongly recommend are Dr. Susan Love's Breast Book and Dr. Peter Pressman and Dr. Yashar Hirshaut's Breast Cancer—The Complete Guide. Breast Book is broad enough to give a solid overview with good specificity on all aspects regarding breasts and breast cancer. It is 683 pages, with a very good glossary that helped tune me in to the nomenclature of cancer. While it doesn't cover each topic in too much detail, it does break down pretty much all of the important topics relative to breasts and breast cancer using language that is concise and remarkably easy to read. Breast Cancer—The Complete Guide covers all of the medical and technical issues surrounding breast cancer in a non-intimidating way that is easy to digest, with a specific focus on the treatment of breast cancer from a surgical and oncological point-of-view. The writing is very crisp as it covers in scientific terms the medical and surgical aspects of breast cancer, while also considering its emotional, cosmetic and financial sides.

After coming home from Barnes & Noble, I put on my running clothes, stretched and took a long run in Central Park. Following my run, Cathy went out with the boys as I sank into my favorite chair to read. I didn't stop until the next morning.

My afternoon and evening's read was not encouraging, in part because we had just determined that Cathy's family tree showed a preponderance of breast cancer. Page 232 of Dr. Love's *Breast Book* states, "if you are a Jewish woman, younger than forty with breast cancer [Cathy is both], there is a 33% chance that you are a carrier of the BRCA-1 gene." This genetic marker significantly elevates the chances of a woman getting breast and/or ovarian cancer. Since the book couldn't further quantify the chances of being a carrier based on Cathy's family tree, I assumed that, based on the preponderance of cancers from her father's family, Cathy was a carrier. With that, it stated clearly that Cathy, as a genetic carrier of the BRCA-1 or BRCA-2 genes would have a 1 to 2 percent chance per year of developing a secondary "primary" cancer. This means that she could develop breast cancer in her left breast unrelated to the cancer in her right breast. This meant not only a potential second surgery later, but also another risk of metastasis, doing chemo twice, and a lifetime of dread. I didn't need a calculator because the math here was shockingly simple: Cathy at thirty eight should be able to live forty two more years if the cancer didn't kill her. This nominally would mean that she would have a 63% chance (the average of 1 and 2%, 1.5 times 42) of developing breast cancer in her other breast.

Medically, it appeared that removing both breasts was the right thing to do. Yet, from an emotional standpoint, it was hard to digest. Forty-eight hours earlier, Cathy had no concerns whatsoever about her health. Fortunately, we learned from our physician interviews that the results of reconstructive surgery are significantly better from an aesthetic perspective when the plastic surgeon can do both breasts at the same time. Invariably, when they do only one breast, it is often difficult to match the new with the old. It is also more challenging to match the nipple and posture of the newly reconstructed breast to the surviving breast, which means, the plastic surgeon has to do some cosmetic work on the surviving breast as well. Plus, the size of the new breast is largely governed by the size of the remaining breast, which seems obvious unless you think of this in the context of redoing your breasts from a purely cosmetic standpoint. If you reconstruct both breasts you have significant latitude in defining their size, shape and posture. Very few women ask for their new breasts to be smaller than the ones they lost (and no husband I have ever spoken to has made such a request).

After a night of reading, by 5:00 Sunday morning our surgical outlook became clearer—Cathy would need to have bilateral mastectomies. It would be safer oncologically, better long-term psychologically and more aesthetically pleasing to both of us. Sitting in my living room before the sun came up, I knew that breaking this news to Cathy was going to be hard. I had no idea what her reaction would be, as two days earlier we both cried after learning she would lose one breast.

I called Cathy's gynecologist, Jean Chin, and had her paged. She was not too pleased to be awakened on a Sunday morning before dawn, but she called me back pretty quickly and immediately focused on Cathy's medical needs and helping us make smart choices.

I recall two things from our conversation that morning. First, Jean agreed that Cathy was definitely a carrier of the BRCA-1 gene. Upon telling her about Cathy's family tree, she said, "Save your money on the genetic testing; she is a carrier." The other memorable part of this pre-dawn conversation was my comparing curing Cathy's cancer to building or remodeling a house. I complained to Jean that I felt like I was the general contractor, and that each individual doctor along the way was merely a subcontractor.

I actually became angry that I was making discoveries and coming to conclusions when I felt a doctor should have been doing this. In my naiveté,
I thought that Jean should have been the one to interpret all of this information for us, as well as recommend a battery of physicians who could
"tell" us the proper treatment. After all, she wasn't just a trusted, respected and highly educated New York City gynecologist—she was Cathy's
trusted, respected and highly educated New York City gynecologist. I
make my living as a commercial real estate broker. My education isn't
grounded in science, much less medicine, so why on Earth should I have
been the one to do the family tree, find and read the right books, discov-
er that my wife was a carrier of the BRCA-1 gene, and then figure out the
type of major life-altering surgery she would need forty eight hours after
learning the very basics about breast cancer?

To her credit, Jean was terrific in this part of the conversation; she didn't
waste time dealing with my frustrations and wasn't intimidated with the
way I communicated them. She answered my questions right there on the
spot, agreed with me about the need to do bilateral mastectomies, and
encouraged me to keep working along the lines I had been working as she
knew that an educated patient and spouse would make better decisions
that would enhance the prospects of survival. Jean also made it clear that
we could call her anytime, and that she would be there for us as needed
during any aspect of this process. She has been true to her word. She did-
n't take us by the hand, but was there whenever we had a question and
wanted her opinion.

The reason that I felt like some general contractor was because I discovered that medical care in the world of cancer is completely fragmented.
The internists, cardiologists and gynecologists who know their patients
best may be involved in the diagnosis of cancer, but have little or even
nothing to do with treating it. There is a handoff to radiologists, surgeons
and oncologists who patients and their spouses generally don't know or

trust. They don't have time to develop a meaningful rapport with any of the physicians involved in cancer treatment, yet they are forced to choose a surgery team and hospital as well as make surgical and treatment decisions, often times with conflicting advice, under great time pressure and with enormous stakes.

Those first few days for me were a blur of medical realities—hard facts and decisions—getting to the right doctors and accepting our new life. For Cathy, these few days were a blur of emotion and hard work as she prepared herself for the rigors of surgery and the reality that she might die.

When I told her that I had called her gynecologist and that we determined she would need bilateral mastectomies, Cathy replied, "That's fine. I don't want to live the rest of my life with the constant fear of this coming back anyway." She then asked me if I wanted coffee. No tears, protests, pity or any other reaction that I would have expected. Her ability to immediately accept her fate took my breath away.

Cathy spent a fair amount of time alone, taking long walks, and thinking. Always thinking. She'd come home and make lists and lists. The lists were an inventory of everything she did for Brandon, Ryan, and me and a playbook of how these things should be handled in the event she wouldn't be around to do them. Some were mundane, like reminding me to scratch Brandon's back each night before he fell asleep, or how much syrup Ryan liked in his "chocolate milky." Others were more serious, like her perspective on Brandon's learning disabilities and her informed feelings on remediating those problems. Cathy tried to put her life on autopilot because her overriding concern was not for herself, but for protecting her family— her kids and me. This process helped her adapt to the reality that her life would never be the same again. The enormity of these lists intimidated me; they showed me how much I didn't know about Cathy's life.

The next week was immensely productive. We were better informed and less emotional about confronting Cathy's cancer when we saw the surgeon from New York Hospital who was recommended to us by Barbara Edelstein. He was smart, gentle and extremely well spoken as he clearly communicated the surgical realities of Cathy's tumor and described carefully how surgery and reconstruction would work. We were inclined to use him as our surgeon because of his reputation, kindness and professionalism. He was totally prepared for us when we walked into his office, having reviewed the mammogram films, and he was prepared to explain what they meant and what the surgical outlook would be for us. In a gentle way, he was all business.

Cathy and I were really impressed with this doctor and knew of the outstanding reputation of the reconstructive plastic surgeon with whom he partnered. He was both surprised and impressed that even though we understood that the tumor was only in Cathy's right breast, our preference—as a result of our own research—was to remove both breasts. Our hour together was spent in front of his light box, learning about Cathy's breasts and the tumor while he answered our questions and described how he would operate and how reconstruction would work. Again, my gut feeling was to use him, as he, also indicated that he could perform the surgery within the next week. I was still very focused on getting this thing out of Cathy as soon as possible, but this time I was more reserved with my comments. I did tell Cathy, and she agreed that this surgeon was very impressive. But we stayed with our plan and met another surgeon, Dr. Alexandra Heerdt of Memorial Sloan Kettering Cancer Center, the next day.

Getting an appointment with Dr. Heerdt, just before Christmas and on short notice, was tough. Alexandra was unlike anyone either of us had ever met. She's an attractive, warm, young (thirty seven years old) surgeon with a reputation for brilliance. She graduated college and medical school in five years (but probably could have done it in three). She has three children under the age of seven, a long commute into the city, works out every day and has a very full schedule between operating on patients and seeing them in her office at the hospital. The other surgeons and operating room nurses at the hospital all raved about her work. When I met her and learned a bit about her background, I was inclined to ask when she found time to sleep.

Because we had already accepted the fact that we would need to remove both breasts and learned so much more about breast cancer and surgery from our last appointment, our forty-five minutes with Alexandra were fact-filled and super-informative. She had the advantage of going last among the surgeons that we interviewed—at that point, we were all business and had educated ourselves by speaking with no less than six physicians and reading over one thousand pages on breasts and breast cancer.

Alexandra walked into the room completely prepared, was economical with her words and was an excellent listener. We wrote out our questions beforehand, but waited to ask them until after Dr. Heerdt spoke to us. While listening and responding to our questions, she looked Cathy squarely in the eyes and held her hand. She confidently expressed that the surgical outlook was very promising, which was comforting to us, but she didn't sugarcoat anything she said. My friend Mary Ann Tighe referred to Memorial Sloan Kettering Cancer Center (MSKCC) as the house of miracles. She was familiar with MSKCC because her husband, Dr. David Hidalgo, before moving to private practice, had been head of reconstructive surgery there. Together, when I called them for advice, they gently convinced me that MSKCC was where we needed to be as it would be the best platform to enhance our prospects of disease-free survival through surgery, chemotherapy, and monitoring afterward.

About halfway through our consultation, I felt that Dr. Heerdt was going to be Cathy's surgeon for many reasons, not the least of which was that MSKCC is an aggressive place. Cathy's pathology report indicated that she had an infiltrating tumor. Simply put, her cancer was aggressive, had already moved beyond the ducts in her breast and was likely fast moving. It was obvious to me that we needed a compassionate surgeon who was also aggressive and from a cutting-edge cancer center. The expression "fight fire with fire" kept going through my head. Our preparation for this meeting allowed us not only to ask the right questions, but also to be better listeners. We listened with our intellects, not just our hearts. Having seen first-hand how fragmented cancer care can be, we liked the idea that at MSKCC we could easily move between surgery and oncology, then onto plastics and whatever other cancer-related specialties we would need.

Without even looking at me for guidance, Cathy told Alexandra that she was going to be her surgeon and that we wanted to schedule a surgery date. This was another example of Cathy's ultimate leadership role in making choices. While we had the same goals, she was the patient and had final say on all matters. We asked Alexandra if she could work with Dr. Joseph Disa as our reconstructive surgeon (even though we hadn't yet met him). We wanted Dr. Disa largely because he trained under David Hidalgo while David was still at MSKCC. Dr. Disa is also considered an outstanding reconstructive surgeon who is conscientious, accessible and a very nice person. Alexandra often worked with Joe and said that it should be no problem.

We were pleased and relieved. We walked out of Dr. Heerdt's office and over to a scheduling desk, where a young man scheduled our surgery for January 20—more than a month away. Scheduling surgery was tricky because we needed a date that both surgeons operated, were free and when there was an available OR (operating room) slot. We faced a four-week delay due to the Christmas holiday and a plastic surgery conference in Hawaii that Joe Disa would be attending in early January. We found our team, but had a date that really didn't feel right. Still, we were so relieved to have a team and hospital in place that we didn't resist the late surgery date on the spot. This was my mistake because Cathy was immediately ill at ease when she heard the date, but I was slow to react. There was a line of other people waiting to see the scheduler, so instead of digging in and pressing for an earlier date, I demurred and lead Cathy out of there. As we left the hospital, Cathy plainly said that she only needed a week or two to prepare for surgery and that waiting would serve no productive purpose whatsoever. She was calm, firm and correct. How could I have walked out of there without fighting as hard as I could to get an earlier date? For a moment, I had taken my eyes off the ball.

That weekend, we left our apartment and headed to our weekend home in Westhampton Beach, about eighty miles east of the city, for some solitude as a family. We were drained, but knew that we had to steel ourselves for a period of great uncertainty and pain. It was a miserably cold and gray Sunday morning, and we ordinarily would not have gone to our weekend home. There, at the breakfast table we decided that notwithstanding the upcoming ordeal in our lives, we would take our Christmas vacation in California the following week as planned. We then focused on the logistics of surgery and of Cathy's immediate term recovery. Over a second cup of coffee, while Brandon and Ryan watched TV in the next room, we discussed our feelings about the time period between diagnosis and surgery, and listed all of the reasons why we felt a surgery date of January 20 was intolerable.

In the middle of our conversation, the phone rang. It was my oldest son's mother, Inbal, calling from her home in Israel. She, too, never calls me early in the morning, so when I heard her voice, I tensed up. Our son Or, a—then nineteen-year-old paratrooper in the Israeli Army, had been in a car accident while on his day off. Our phone conversation went like this:

Inbal (voice shaking): Mark there has been a terrible accident.
Me: Is he alive? Has Or been killed?

Inbal (hesitating for a few seconds because the intensity in my voice must have surprised her): No.

Me: He's been killed?

Inbal: No. He's been badly injured in a car accident and will need to have surgery on his knee and stitches in his face.

Me (numbed with relief): What happened? Tell me everything... I'll be there tomorrow.

I had just spoken to Or the day before and we had a heart to heart talk as I explained what Cathy was up against. Even though we were on a phone and half a world apart, I could feel his steadiness and love when he told me, "I'm sorry, Dad. Be as strong as you can be." Now he was in the hospital and would need to have surgery to reconstruct his kneecap and close up some of his facial cuts.

My already frayed nerves were now shot. I had always considered myself a tough guy, but now my mettle was being tested and I clearly remember being unsure that I would be up to the task of holding everything together. Just over a week earlier, I was "focused" on finishing a few year-end transactions, my Christmas vacation, and perhaps correcting my slice on the golf course. Now my concerns were ranging from oncology to orthopedics on two continents, with two of the four people I love most in the world.

We immediately drove back to the city and that evening with Cathy's support and encouragement, I found myself on a plane to Israel. Since it was still Sunday, I didn't have the opportunity to even try to change her surgery date. My immediate concern was to make sure that Or had a very competent orthopedic surgeon, stay with him until that surgery was completed, and then fly home to try to schedule an earlier date for Cathy's surgery. After that, I would fly to California to make the last three days of our family vacation.

I took off on a dark and rainy night from Newark Liberty Airport and landed in Tel Aviv on a dark, rainy night. I drove two hours in rush-hour traffic to the hospital where the ambulance had taken my son. When I saw him lying bruised and cut up in his hospital bed, I held him tight. He whispered into my ear, "Sorry, dad, I know you didn't need this now." I didn't want to release him because if I did, he would have seen that I was crying. The stress of the last ten days combined with sleep deprivation had made me emotional, so instead of moving, I held him with my cheek on his for about two minutes.

The Army and Or's mother arranged for a highly experienced and skilled orthopedic surgeon to reconstruct Or's kneecap the next day. After the surgery, the surgeon told me that he was highly optimistic that Or would make a relatively full recovery, which he expected would take between four and six months. I had conflicting emotions about this—while I was upset that Or was hurt, I was also somewhat relieved that he wouldn't be engaged in any high-risk military activities for the next few months.

While sitting at my son's bedside, Inbal arranged for her best friend Aya to call me on the cell phone that I rented at the airport. Aya had undergone bilateral mastectomies and adjuvant chemotherapy two years earlier, while she, her husband Fonti and their two young children were living in Boston. In a one-hour conversation, I learned a tremendous amount from both Aya and Fonti, including how Aya's surgery was far easier than the course of chemotherapy she underwent. At this point, I didn't know that Cathy would require chemotherapy, and was unfamiliar with the drugs prescribed for the different types of chemo.

On my way to the airport at the end of my visit, I drove my rented car to Jerusalem, about an hour away, and found my way to the Western Wall of the Temple Mount. There, Joshua originally built a Temple for God, which was destroyed and rebuilt by Solomon, as chronicled in *The Book of Numbers*. Actually, the Temple has been destroyed several times, but the Western Wall has always been, and remains, the holiest spot for my religion. Notwithstanding that it was the height of the "Intifada," and Jerusalem was eerily empty, I was determined to pray there for Cathy, Or, Brandon and Ryan. In a freezing rain, I stood next to the Wall, the Kotel, and prayed a heartfelt prayer of thanksgiving that Or had survived his car accident and that Cathy's cancer could be cured. I asked God to cure her, and to give me the strength and wisdom to support her and my entire family.

On my overnight flight back to New York, I went from focusing on my son's knee to my wife's cancer and the necessary logistics for getting her cured. With a pen and the back of a napkin, I did some calculating.

We discovered that Cathy had breast cancer on December 12. Our surgery date was January 20—a full forty days later. Cathy and I became consumed with the thought that by waiting for a convenient date for the two surgeons, we were wasting the benefit of the early detection that was afforded by mammography. Waiting to remove an aggressive, fast-growing tumor once we knew it needed to be removed seemed completely illogical. We were confident that we had the right surgeons and hospital, but we were equally certain that we had the wrong date.

I instinctively knew that any discussions with a surgeon or oncologist would be uneven and that medically, I couldn't persuade them into feeling that Cathy would be harmed by waiting an extra two weeks for her surgery

31

if they didn't already feel that way. I did, however, construct an unassailable argument that the doctors couldn't refute; one, which centered on the emotional toll that waiting, would take on both Cathy and myself. If we accepted the later surgery date and Cathy died, I would be tortured the rest of my life and Cathy would die with a horrible sense of guilt. Furthermore, the anxiety caused by the delayed surgery date would be emotionally and physically destructive to both of us, so much so that we were prepared to revisit our decision to seek treatment at MSKCC.

The day I returned from Israel, I went to see Lisa Lieberman, the head of the Breast Center at MSKCC. Although I didn't have an appointment, she graciously received me in her office, and I communicated, in very straightforward language, the argument I had crafted on the plane flight home. I added that while we wanted to use MSKCC for both surgery and oncology, I was inclined to go to another hospital for the surgery if they could do it sooner. Lisa must have seen a pitifully tired, jet-lagged and stressed-out husband who was at his wits end with concern for his wife. She assured me that she would try to change the dates and rework the surgery schedules of both surgeons, but that I needed to give her some time.

I called David Hidalgo later that day and explained the problems I was having with re-scheduling Cathy's surgery. Throughout his career, David has used his very tactical mind to guide people through unimaginable medical problems. He listened to my approach and suggested that it might just work; MSKCC wouldn't want to lose a patient to another hospital simply because they couldn't accommodate them with an appropriate surgery date. I suspect that David then called one or both surgeons on my behalf and prevailed upon them to move heaven and Earth and perform our surgery earlier. I will never know for sure because he wasn't helping me for "the credit," but because he is genuinely a caring man.

The next day I found my weary body in Los Angeles. Lisa Lieberman called my cell phone that afternoon to happily advise us that the surgery date was changed to January 8 at 7:00 A.M. My sense of relief was overwhelming— we finally had the right team and the right hospital doing the right procedure on the best possible date. I was pretty drained at this point, but knew that we hadn't even reached the starting line and had a long way to go. Now our focus went toward getting ready for surgery.

CHAPTER 3
TALKING TO YOUR YOUNG CHILDREN ABOUT MOMMY'S CANCER

For me, one of the hardest parts of dealing with Cathy's cancer was protecting our children from the trauma of their mother's ordeal. I wanted to be able to tell our kids that their mommy was going to be fine and that everything would be okay. But the truth was that when Cathy was first diagnosed, I didn't know if everything would be fine—and I didn't want to erode our kids' trust by first painting a rosy picture and then having to cast dark shadows on it later.

Prior to Cathy's surgery, while I was immersed in the strategy of how to best attack her cancer, my thoughts constantly drifted to my sons in that I wondered how I might raise them alone if Cathy didn't survive. I wanted to push the image of myself as a widower raising two young boys out of my head, but soon realized that this was impossible. I had to be practical and prepare myself and my family for whatever was in our future. Cathy and I decided that first and foremost, we needed to determine how to properly insulate our sons from the effects of her surgery and treatment.

Our boys, Brandon and Ryan, were eight and three years old, respectively, at the time of Cathy's diagnosis. Their half-brother Or is my son, and he and his mother Inbal live in Israel. Although we never married, Inbal is very close with Cathy and myself, so much so that Brandon regards her as his "other mother." While Or loves Cathy and had spent a lot of time with her when he was growing up, my principal concern was now for Brandon and Ryan, who were at very impressionable ages and completely dependent on their mom.

Brandon is a sensitive boy who is drop-dead handsome, intelligent, charismatic and learning disabled. The year before Cathy's diagnosis, Brandon had to leave the private school he was attending because of these disabilities. Upon evaluation, we learned that Brandon couldn't properly process written, multisyllabic words and was profoundly dis-graphic. As the parents of any child with learning disabilities can attest, Brandon was in a tough state emotionally before finding out that his mother had cancer, since he knew that he was different from his friends and classmates, and interpreted that difference as being "stupid." We were finally getting him comfortable with himself and beginning the process of lifting his self-esteem when cancer visited our home. Consequently, Brandon's school life and home life were going to be unsteady at best for the next year. Typically, Cathy would be the one to guide and nurture him through any crisis or problem in his life. Now it would fall disproportionately on me, and I was unsure of my ability to handle it.

Ryan is a super-bright, resilient child who confidently faced the pressures of being a three-year-old and has been Daddy's boy since he was born. In the months before Cathy was diagnosed, Ryan was at a particularly clingy stage of development, not easily separating himself from his mom at nursery school, and he was generally finding his way into our bed in the middle of the night.

Our boys were at impressionable, sensitive times in their lives, and we knew that how we moved through the next twelve months as a family would have a significant impact on their short and long-term emotional development. We realized that while there is no perfect roadmap to deal-ing with your children, since each specific illness is different and chil-dren's ages and needs vary greatly, there are excellent reference materials and well-informed experts, both of which can be very helpful. We listened to the advice of mental health professionals as well as that which we obtained from several books and the reference materials that I picked up at MSKCC. We also paid close attention to our gut feelings and I reflected back on my own personal experience as a young boy who had to deal with my own mother's breast cancer.

When I was seven years old in 1969, my mother was diagnosed with the disease and underwent a "radical" mastectomy. My mom, Jeannette Weiss, was a beautiful thirty seven-year-old woman (she is now a beautiful seventy one-year-old woman), raising three small children in a modest home in a working-class neighborhood on Long Island. During a routine physical she received some very disturbing news: she had a suspicious lump on one of her breasts that needed to be removed. She was told that in all likelihood it was benign and that she shouldn't be concerned. She was also told that they wouldn't know for sure until a biopsy was performed, which at that time could only be done through surgery. If a malignancy were found, her breast would need to be "removed" as well.

My mom was raised in Cairo, Egypt and in Paris, France, and as a child was inculcated with the notion that doctors knew all and were generally not to be questioned. She was ill prepared for "the worst" because her doctors didn't want her to worry "unnecessarily." She woke up from her surgery and knew instantly that she had been, in her words, "mutilated." She had no frame of reference for what had happened or what would happen to her. Years later, as she related her feelings to me, she remembered praying, "God, please let me live long enough to raise my children." The denial, anger and betrayal she felt was immense because she thought she was going to wake up from surgery with only a small scar on her breast. Instead, she woke up with no nipple, no breast, and fewer lymph nodes and axillary muscles. To this day, her surgery is defined by a long vertical scar where her breast had been. She was basically left alone to start a process of recovering from a disease that she didn't understand, wasn't prepared to face, thought would kill her, couldn't talk about and really couldn't define for herself because of the lack of published information and society's inhibition at that time for words like cancer and breast.

It wasn't until 1977 that surgeons started to utilize a two-step process of biopsy followed a few weeks later, (if necessary), with a mastectomy. These few precious weeks gave women and their husbands and children time to prepare for the gravity of what they were about to face. Today, many biopsies are done using an ultrasound-guided needle to aspirate the tumor. This technology simply wasn't around for my mom in the seventies. Needless to say, she was sad and angry, and had few (if any) outlets for her anger.

I tried to recall what discernible recollections I had that were specific to her operation. Sadly, I have few because I didn't know anything that was going on with my mother. You see, I wasn't told that she had breast cancer until I was sixteen years old, which to this day seems incredible to me. I can't believe my parents were able to keep this illness such a secret. As a young child, I lived in a house that had much sadness and pain, and I had no idea why. I was, however, probably more fortunate than my three-year-old brother, Paul. I was at school most days, while he was home during the time of my mother's physical and emotional convalescence.

I feel certain that if we had been told the truth, even at our young ages, we would have understood and accepted the uncertainty, and actually been helpful to my mother. But I've never questioned my parents' love for us, and I know that their instinct was to protect my brothers and me from the fear and pain of an unpredictable, and potentially lethal disease. The common wisdom in the sixties was to keep children in the dark about cancer—or anything bad for that matter. From where I sit now, I believe that children should be informed and involved in varying degrees, depending on their age and level of maturity.

While planning the best way to deal with Brandon and Ryan, I called Paul, who now lives in Florida. I wanted to see if he had any recollections about Mom's illness, but because he was so young at the time, he didn't. It was really most unfortunate because my younger brother might have helped me relate to the way Ryan might interpret events. Paul did support the concept of informing Brandon and Ryan, but wasn't sure how much information they would be able to handle.

I then called my older brother Gary and asked him what he remembered about Mom's surgery and its aftermath. Gary was eight-years-old when my mother was diagnosed and treated, and he remembered a lot. He recounted a story for me that I only vaguely remember. It was early in 1970. There was plenty of snow on the ground, and he and I were enjoying a one-on-one snowball fight, which I was losing badly. I called for a truce, to which Gary agreed, as he was always very fair with me. During this armistice, I threw a snowball at Gary and hit him in the head, which infuriated him so much that he gave chase with a freshly made snowball. Fearing his retribution, I ran to take cover in the house, knowing it would provide sanctuary from snowballs. Gary, unimpressed with my notion of sanctuary, threw the snowball at me while I was opening the side door, and it followed me through the door and landed with a wet, messy thud on the kitchen floor. Gary vividly recalled this entire incident because my mother reacted so hysterically and became so angry that she began to hyperventilate.

In telling me about this incident, Gary pointed out that as an eight-year-old, he felt that he had caused our mother's total distress that day. Only now can I visualize my young mother sitting alone at the kitchen table during a rare quiet moment in our house with a cup of coffee. She was probably sitting there trying to process all that had recently happened to her when she was startled by that snowball. This incident was traumatic for Gary, as he carried around the guilt and pain of causing my mother so much agony. The night I called him for advice, we discussed how much we would have benefited if we were given some context for my mother's anger and pain. It would have freed us from blaming ourselves, and in fact allowed us to try to help our mother. This, in turn, would have been helpful to her and to us. Gary was emphatic in urging me to tell Or, Brandon and Ryan as soon as possible.

When I got off the phone with Gary, I thought about one of the only clear recollections I have of my mother's experience with cancer. I remember being with my dad and Gary, playing in Carl Schulz Park, across the street from Doctor's Hospital in New York City. I remember crossing the street going into the hospital and seeing my mother lying in her hospital bed, crying intensely. As I recall her face now, it had the emotion of Debra Winger's face in the movie *Terms of Endearment*, on the day she said goodbye to her children for the last time. I didn't understand my mother's pain then. I just remember feeling very helpless. At that time, a cancer diagnosis was often a death sentence; there was no chemotherapy, and surgical practices were not terribly refined. Early detection was just a matter of luck. In her postoperative confusion, my mother probably felt like she was going to die. Only now can I appreciate the strain that must have placed on my father.

Another recollection I have is much more vivid. I was a sixteen-year-old watching TV in our den one evening when my mother came in to talk to me. My aunt, her sister Adeline, also had breast cancer and had just undergone surgery. I told Mom that I was concerned about my aunt and where her cancer might lead. It was then that she said, "Many women have survived cancer."

I immediately replied, "Like who?"

Finally, she dropped the bombshell. "Me. I did, in 1969."

I looked at her and asked, "But you didn't have your breast removed? Right?" She then told me that she had.

I remember hugging and trying to comfort her and telling her how much I loved her. It's funny, but I was instinctively doing for my mother then what I know I could have done for her as a child, had I been told.

I was in a funk for a few weeks after that conversation with my mom. I specifically remember sitting on the team bus one day after a lacrosse game. I played really poorly, but I didn't care; I was sad and depressed about my mother's cancer even though it was 1978, a full nine years after her surgery. Coach Schiller spoke to me on the bus about my poor play, but I couldn't process any of what he said. I was focused on my feelings of parental vulnerability and guilt in not having been able to support and defend my mom during the previous nine years. I was also angry with myself for all of the hard times I gave her as a child. How could I have never helped her with the laundry? Why did I have to be asked twice to carry in the groceries? I kept thinking, How could they have not told me earlier?

My parents probably didn't tell us in part because they didn't want us to feel an obligation to do things differently than regular kids in regular households. Gary and Paul probably had a tougher experience with my mother's illness—at least relative to mine—because Gary was older and remembered more, while Paul couldn't escape a household of pain for even a few hours a day. The three of us would have benefited if my parents sat us down and explained to us that "the doctors found a disease called cancer in Mommy's breast and were able to cure her by removing the disease in the operating room. It hurts Mommy a little, but she will get better very soon. She might be sad for a little while because while she gets better it might be hard for her to carry you and to make all of your favorite foods." This would have given us an ability to process what was happening, as well as a reason not to blame ourselves for any sadness or anger that we saw in our mother. Gary and I certainly would have been able to deal with this. Paul was a smart child and would have taken from this explanation more than my parents could have reasonably expected. A modicum of information presented to us while we were young would have spared us a shock in our teenage years.

I recently asked my parents why they didn't tell us about what my mother went through when she was going through it. As I suspected, they asked me to consider the times in which they were living their nightmare. In 1969, the Women's Movement as we know it hadn't been born. I bring this up because one of the spectacular successes of the Women's Movement was the publicizing of women's health issues—especially breast cancer.

Before women started advocating for themselves, people just didn't talk openly about women's health issues. Society was so closed in the sixties that Americans still thought Lucy and Ricky slept in separate beds. Cancer was a word that was whispered and considered synonymous with "certain death." People also didn't speak publicly about any part of a women's anatomy—especially parts that had to do with sexuality. It was also a time when women were considered too emotionally fragile to handle the gravity of real-life problems. One of the physicians treating my mother actually suggested to my father that they concoct a story so that my mother wouldn't realize she had a serious life-threatening condition. Fortunately, my father rejected this idiotic advice.

It wasn't until the seventies, when Betty Ford and Happy Rockefeller went public about their battles with breast cancer, that the subject became a widespread topic of "acceptable" conversation. In the eighties, Olivia Newton-John, Sandra Day O'Connor and Nancy Reagan followed them, which did our society a tremendous service; they provided both men and women with knowledge about a potentially deadly disease that did not discriminate based on race or social standing. This knowledge empow-ered hundreds of thousands of women to deal with breast cancer before it dealt with them.

Every bookstore today has lots to read on breast cancer, from the scien-tific to the emotional aspects of the disease. There are support groups everywhere, and we are inundated with public service messages encour-aging mammography and other forms of early detection. Women wear the twisted pink ribbon as a sign of pride for having survived this malicious disease and in support of more research. In 1969 and 1970, there were no such things. Society's unspoken advice to women with breast cancer was to go die quietly, so in the context of those times, it is unlikely that Gary, Paul and I would have been told that "mommy had breast cancer." Sad for us, sad for my mother and sad for my father, as he had to shoulder a big burden on his own. While society was more closed in the 1960's than today, cancer was also a different disease in that there was no such thing as adjuvant therapy. Chemotherapy hadn't been invented yet, which meant that the survival rates for people with cancer were considerably lower. Furthermore, early detection was not nearly as prevalent then as it is now. By the time a woman went to a surgeon, there was already a high probability that the cancer had metastasized. Today, breast cancer is usu-ally detected before it has metastasized.

In the context of those closed times, it would have been unrealistic to expect my parents to be open and truthful with us. As soon as Cathy was diagnosed, I became almost fanatical to learn as much as I could about the disease. I needed to empower myself with information so that I could be a supportive, effective husband and partner in fighting cancer. I want-ed to help Cathy intelligently question physicians and choose the right team to get us through this ordeal. While somewhat fragmented, the information on breast cancer is out there and accessible (provided you stay away from the Internet, as I mentioned earlier). My parents relied 100 percent on the advice of their doctors, in part because they were raised to think doctors are a cut above the general population, but also because there was a dearth of published information on breast cancer. Their basic lack of knowledge about the disease made it very difficult to break it down into child-sized bites for Gary, Paul and me. The only logical thing for them to do was "protect" us by not telling us anything. Keeping someone in the dark was regarded as a way of safeguarding him or her from unnecessary fear and worry.

While we were inclined, based on our gut feelings and past experiences, to inform Brandon and Ryan about what we were facing, we also made certain to get advice on this topic from mental health professionals. One of the great things about living in New York City is that it feels like there are two million mental health professionals treating New York's eight million residents. We availed ourselves to the opinions of three different psychiatrists on how to deal with our kids. They were pretty uniform in imparting their advice of informing and empowering children with balanced and hopeful information. This affirmed our instincts and supported my own feelings based on my childhood experiences, which were fortified by the blunt observation of respected psychiatrist Dr. Abba Borowich. When I asked him how I could protect my boys from the stress of their mother's illness, he suggested hopeful candor, but also told me, "Mark, your children will grow up very fast with this. You cannot protect them to the degree you would like."

Within a few days, Cathy and I had soul-searched, researched, and consulted with others until we finally, believed we had enough information to draft a series of points, which we used to guide ourselves in dealing with her cancer and our kids. I expounded on each of these points and listed them here because I realize that a lot of parents facing a similar situation might find them helpful:

- Be honest and forthright with your children. They can handle more than you think and will benefit immeasurably from understanding what is going on in their home. If you don't tell them what is happening, they will assume the worst and their assumption can be much more gruesome than reality.

● Put a positive upbeat spin on any news that you give them—"Mommy is really sick, but we found a way that will make her better and we are so happy about that," goes a long way.

● Tell your children that cancer is not contagious and that nothing they did caused Mommy's cancer. Children are generally taught that sickness (colds and flu) are contagious and have heard things like "Billy was here and was sneezing, and now all of us are sick."

● Prepare your children before they hear something incredibly stupid from an adult or something unintentionally hurtful or damaging from another child. Cathy and I have heard of countless times when the child of a woman with cancer learns about it from another child or that child's parent. Ironically, it is the parents more often than their children who say these hurtful things.

● Find the right supporting materials to clarify any information that you impart to your children. My favorite book was called *Kemo Shark* about a shark that was invented by scientists and eats all of the bad cells that make mommy sick. Unfortunately, some of the good cells look like bad cells, and Kemo Shark hurts those cells, but doesn't kill them. This damage to the good cells is called side effects! I read this fourteen-page story to Brandon and Ryan while Cathy was in the hospital. They both absorbed it and learned a tremendous amount from it. Imagine being a child and having to digest the concept that there is a medicine that makes you really sick so that it can make you better. Pretty confusing!

- Find outlets so that they can be away from home during the ghastly days after surgery and chemo. A trip to Grandma and Grandpa's house during these tough days is generally good for everyone—including Grandma and Grandpa, who want so badly to help.
- Surround your children with comforting people and things. Don't let negative people anywhere near your house or your children. Events in your wife's medical care may be bleak, though upbeat people will somehow make you and your kids feel upbeat.
- Involve your children's teachers and principals in your support system. You will be pleasantly surprised at the levels of support and compassion from your children's educators. Don't assume that they know very much about cancer. Explain it to them, from surgery to chemo to the effects of both. My children's teachers and principals were terrific. We sent them copies of Kemo Shark so that they could relate to the materials we used to help inform our children.
- Constantly reassure your children that they will be OK! Kids need to be told that they will be well and not get sick like mommy because kids are basically selfish. Their main fear is "Am I going to be OK?" Well, nothing reassured my kids more than hearing from their dad, "Mommy is going to be OK, I am going to be OK, Brandon and Or are going to be OK, and Ryan will be OK! Everybody is going to be OK."

We decided that the time was right to speak to the boys when I caught up with Cathy, Brandon and Ryan in California. We did the Disneyland thing a few hours after I arrived. I was so jet lagged that I didn't even know what day it was, but Cathy and I felt that the trip to Disneyland would help lighten the magnitude of the news we were about to deliver. On the ride there, we had a family meeting in the car. That meant everyone gave their complete attention—radios and Game Boys were turned off. Our carefully choreographed conversation with Brandon and Ryan went as follows:

Cathy: Boys, we have something very important to talk about.

Talking to Your Children About Mommy's Cancer

Me: Mommy has something called "the curable cancer." This is a disease that is inside Mommy.

Cathy: But we are really happy because we found the best doctors in the world, right in New York City, who said they could remove the disease in a very simple operation.

Me: These great doctors can take the curable cancer out of Mommy.

Ryan: Will they take it out of Mommy's mouth?

Brandon: Ryan, don't be silly. Will they?

Me: Actually, boys, it is in Mommy's breast. They will cut it out without hurting Mommy, but she will have to go into the hospital.

Brandon: How long will she be in the hospital?

Cathy: Just a few days.

Ryan: Will they give you ice cream, like Curious George?

Cathy: Yes, Ryan, they will. What flavor should I have?

Ryan: Vanilla would be good.

Brandon: Can I play my Game Boy now?

Me: Sure. If you have any questions about this, let us know. We'll be at Disneyland in half an hour.

Kids need time to process information. We were relieved that we started the process of informing our kids in an upbeat way. Later that week, Brandon asked Cathy plenty of questions. I was thankful that he had the open type of relationship with his mother and that he could speak his mind and heart freely. I assumed that Ryan wasn't all that interested or had hit his saturation point for information. That was, until the morning after Cathy's surgery. I came out of the shower and was about to dress and go to the hospital and found Ryan in my room. Looking cute in his blue- and white striped pajamas, he very naturally started this conversation:

Ryan: Daddy, did the doctors wash the bloody knife after they cut Mommy's booby?"

Me: Yes, Ryan, they did. The doctors are very clean. Mommy likes that.
Ryan: Me, too. I want Mommy to make me chocolate milky.

Me: I'll do it. Mommy won't be home for a few days because she is getting better at the hospital.

Ryan: Did the doctors get all of the cancer out of Mommy?

Me: Yes, they did.

Ryan: How do you know they didn't forget some?

Me: Because we were lucky to get the best doctors in the world, and they told me they got it all!

This was our conversation on January 9, 2003. Not a day goes by when I don't hope that I was telling Ryan the truth.

CHAPTER 4

SURGERY—IT'S NOT AN AMPUTATION

January 8, 2003, surgery day was grueling in every way and isn't a day that I'll forget anytime soon. After a sleepless night, Cathy and I met my mother-in-law Phyllis and my parents at MSKCC at 5:00 A.M. There were lots of people checking in for surgery at that time; in a strange way, it was comforting knowing that what was exceptional for us was routine for MSKCC. The admitting nurse was terrific because she combined a sense of humor and upbeat presence along with a businesslike, professional attitude. After checking us in, she walked us across the hospital to the surgery suite on the fifth floor where they were ready for Cathy. The hospital is sprawling; it occupies a full city block and is a labyrinth because it has grown in several stages over the past forty years. Patients are walked to their destination because they don't want a nervous patient wandering around lost for forty minutes while their surgeon cools his or her heels in the operating room!

After changing into a surgery gown, Cathy was examined by a nurse to make sure she hadn't completely succumbed to the stress of having both sets of parents trying to act calm in the face of cancer surgery, and the unknown outcome that would follow it. Then Cathy and I were led to a small waiting area to wait for Alexandra. I held her hand and prayed; I knew we had done all we could to get to this point, and now things were totally outside of our control. For a person who takes great comfort in being in control, this was terribly unsettling.

Alexandra emerged from two giant doors that were off-limits to anyone except medical personnel and patients. As she greeted us she took Cathy's hand. A surgeon in surgical scrubs anywhere near an operating room has a towering presence, not unlike a soldier in combat fatigues. Alexandra gently promised she would call me during the surgery to let me know how things were going. The way she spoke to me had an undertone that I shouldn't respond or ask any questions, as her focus was on Cathy and the business at hand.

It was time for Cathy to go. I hugged her and told her that I loved her, and then she walked down the hall with Alexandra. My brave wife went with her as if she had no fears or concerns, as if they were walking together as doubles partners about to play a semifinal match at Wimbledon. Serious, but confidant. Here, Cathy was leading by example. We had worked really hard to get to this point, and it was time for me to quite literally step up and be a strong husband and father.

I went to the waiting area where I saw my parents, Phyllis and about ten or twelve friends. My father-in-law didn't come from California because he felt that the last thing Cathy would need during surgery week was to watch her parents argue. They had divorced when Cathy was twelve, but there was still enough personal friction to cause tempers to flare easily. Our day was already several hours old as surgery started at about 7:30 A.M.

By 8:30 A.M., we must have had about twenty friends in the waiting area. Many of Cathy's friends dropped their kids at school and then came straight to MSKCC, which was nice; I never really knew just how loved my wife was until I saw and felt the concern of her many friends.

I knew that Alexandra would call me from the operating room around 8:45 A.M. This call would be to tell me if Cathy's lymph nodes were clear or if the cancer had spread to them. During surgery, Alexandra would examine Cathy's sentinel lymph node and visually determine if it appeared cancerous. If she detected cancer, she would remove at least the first cluster of lymph nodes.

Part of the pre-admission testing process included injecting Cathy's right breast with a special dye in a process known as sentinel mapping, which allowed her surgeon to identify the lymph nodes that had the highest probability of being cancerous based on their proximity to the affected breast. A surgeon can determine which lymph node is the breast's primary "drainer" because the breasts are drained by the lymphatic system. This closest drainer is called the sentinel node because generally (though not always) it is the lymph node that plays the most significant role in draining the breast. If cancer has spread or metastasized, whether locally or regionally, it would first impact the sentinel node. I fully expected Cathy's lymph nodes to be clear since we had detected her cancer early and received no indication from the radiologists and surgeons that they may have been affected.

There are four stages of cancer, with Stage I being the least serious and most contained, and Stage IV, being the most serious and least contained. Any nodal involvement whatsoever would put a woman at Stage II cancer. Another indicator of Stage II is if the tumor is over 2 centimeters in diameter. Since Cathy's tumor was 1.8 centimeters, I was holding out a tremendous amount of hope that she would have no nodal involvement and be classified as Stage I. Stage II has lower survival rates and comes with a significantly more miserable chemotherapy regimen after surgery.

At MSKCC, information is disseminated from the surgeon to the patient's family by paging a designated family member to the day surgery telephone that's behind the reception desk. The surgeon, using a telephone in the operating room, is able to communicate some general news about the surgery as well as the status of the patient. The way the day surgery telephone is positioned gives a family member only a small amount of privacy to speak to a surgeon, and the conversation is designed to last no more than sixty seconds. I knew that when I was called I would only have time to ask one or two questions at best. I planned my questions carefully, but expected the conversation to be upbeat with only good results. I wanted to know if there was nodal involvement and if Alexandra saw anything that caused particular alarm in Cathy. Actually, I wanted confirmation that there was no nodal involvement and that nothing caused the surgery team alarm or concern.

Lymph nodes look like grapes and come in clusters—typically three—which are generally situated under a woman's arm. In addition to draining a woman's breasts after they become engorged immediately before her menstrual cycle, they also serve to drain a woman's arms, hands and fingers from all types of swelling. They are like the body's own natural wetlands by filtering out impurities and fighting infection. If a woman has Stage II cancer and does everything right from surgery to chemotherapy, her chances of disease-free survival could range from 88%-95% as contrasted to Stage I cancer, which carries a disease-free survival range from 92%-98%. In addition to the lower survival rates, Stage II, at MSKCC and most other cancer centers, is treated with several very toxic chemotherapy agents, including a very potent drug called Adriamycin. While I was aware of these facts, I didn't think they would be applicable, as I felt deep down in my gut that Cathy's cancer hadn't spread to her lymph nodes. I knew that once Alexandra called me from the operating room and told me that her nodes were clean, the end of this ordeal would be in sight. My sense of denial was working on overdrive here. I was completely prepared for the news that I wanted so badly to hear.

At 8:55 A.M., I was paged to the day surgery telephone. As I was walking toward the phone, I literally felt my mother-in-law Phyllis pushing past me. Phyllis knew that I was supposed to be the one to take this call, but she couldn't control herself because Cathy was still her baby. I stepped in front of Phyllis and picked up the phone. On the other end of the line, Alexandra immediately said, "Mark, I don't have the best news. I found cancer in Cathy's sentinel lymph node." She then said something else but I couldn't hear her because Phyllis was literally climbing on top of me, trying to hear both sides of the short conversation. I was able to ask Alexandra if she detected any further spread of the cancer beyond the sentinel node. Her answer was no but that we would talk when she finished in about an hour. My first emotion was frustration because I felt that I missed something important in our forty-second conversation. I was also angry with my mother-in-law for following me and interfering, but my anger could just as easily have been my frustration and disappointment at the troubling news.

Phyllis asked me what Alexandra had said as we were walking back toward the waiting area. Here I made a huge mistake; instead of sitting down, out from view of the rest of our contingency, and slowly explaining to Phyllis what the doctor said and what that would likely mean, I kept walking and said, "Cathy's cancer spread to her sentinel lymph node, but we will understand much more in about an hour." All Phyllis heard was "Cathy," "cancer" and "spread." She immediately burst into tears and fell to her knees at exactly the moment the rest of our friends and family saw us. As I looked up, I saw all of our friends (and even the family and friends of other patients who were undergoing surgery at the same time) start to cry.

It was a chain reaction of misery, and I understood how it happened and that I was responsible. My mother-in-law was out of control because she was unprepared for the surgeon's phone call, and she certainly wasn't ready for bad news to be thrust at her so suddenly. Furthermore, she didn't understand the consequence of nodal involvement because I didn't carefully explain it to her right away. I expected that Phyllis wouldn't interfere with my interactions with the doctors, hospital and decision-making in general, so when I became annoyed with her, I selfishly focused on my own disappointment instead of helping Cathy's mother process this tough news.

I was disgusted that I had to face an entire waiting room full of crying people, and wasn't sure what to say. To this day, I wish I had taken a few minutes with Phyllis and calmly walked her through what I just learned; it would have made everything so much easier on her and everyone there that day. I was dealing with my own disappointment because I had foolishly set my expectations only for good news and wasn't prepared for bad. Phyllis put me under so much pressure to restate what Alexandra said that I didn't have time to carefully think through what she said and what it really meant. If I had about two minutes alone, I could have sorted through my sense of disappointment and accepted that Cathy still could have a very strong chance of disease-free survival. Then I could have faced all of our friends and family and put an upbeat spin on everything.

Cathy and I had agreed that if the results of her surgery were glum we would not share that with people, as we didn't want anyone to assume that she would die, or use the number of cancerous lymph nodes as a scorecard for them to consider Cathy's prospects for survival.

So, instead of dealing with anyone, I briefly explained to our friends that the cancer appears not to have been contained, but that we would know much more later. I headed straight to the elevators and went downstairs for a walk. As I left, I asked my mother and Cathy's friend Jill to comfort Phyllis.

Outside, it was twenty degrees and windy, but the biting cold air felt good as I walked around the block twice and processed what I had learned. This walk helped me accept and understand our new reality, and I was then able to go back into the hospital to face our friends and family. I would tell them that there was some nodal involvement and that in keeping with aggressive and conservative medicine, Dr. Heerdt was removing whatever traces of cancerous cells she saw. I would also inform them that I would be spending a few minutes with Dr. Heerdt after the surgery, at which time she would explain what was happening to Cathy and answer my questions.

While I was still disappointed, I was ready to move on and be positive and productive. But at that moment, God gently gave me some much needed perspective. On the elevator ride back up to the fifth floor surgery wing, I must have hit the wrong button—the elevator opened on the third floor instead, and I inadvertently stepped out to find myself on the pediatric cancer floor. I immediately saw a little bald boy, about six-years old, sitting in a wheelchair and being reassured by his parents. His parents were about my age and in their faces was a fear that I'd never seen before. His mother, wearing a maroon cardigan sweater over a black turtleneck, was holding her son's hand with both of hers. I froze for about four seconds as I made eye contact with the boy's father. Instantly I realized how much smaller my problems were than his. I knew that I was on the wrong floor and was immediately grateful that I wasn't with Or, Brandon or Ryan. Suddenly, the fifth floor seemed like a much less terrifying place for me to spend the morning. I turned around slowly and pressed the "up" elevator button and took the next elevator to five.

Just as I was feeling sorry for myself and at the point of being overwrought with frustration and anger about the spread of Cathy's cancer, I saw how lucky I was. My heart literally ached for the parents of that small boy, and to all the parents who had spent the Christmas holiday in a cancer hospital with their child. Because I saw clearly that nothing I was going through compared to the pain felt by that little boy and his parents. I became more sympathetic to Phyllis; it was her daughter in the operating room, not her spouse. I realized then that while January 8, 2003 was horrible for me, it was probably far worse for my mother-in-law.

I got upstairs and reassured everyone that, notwithstanding Phyllis's reaction, the news wasn't terribly dreadful. I also spent a few minutes with my friend, Rabbi David Laine, who pulled me to a private spot and prayed with me. My voice choked with emotion when we prayed, as I realized with amazing clarity that Cathy's life wasn't in Dr. Alexandra Heerdt's hands at all—it was in *God's* hands. These few minutes where I shed a few private tears were immensely cathartic; all of my stress and bottled-up emotions needed to come out, and it was better that they come out quickly so I could move on more easily.

As we finished, I was paged to the same telephone where I had my last disappointing phone call. This time, Phyllis didn't follow me. Instead of a phone call, I was able to sit with Alexandra on a small, uncomfortable blue couch, which was out of sight from Phyllis of our friends. We had a brief and calm discussion about Cathy's surgery. Alexandra explained that when she saw that the sentinel node was cancerous, she removed it as well as the entire nearest cluster of lymph nodes. A cluster typically contains ten-twelve nodes and, following her surgeon's instinct, Alexandra wanted to send all of the nodes to pathology for a full work-up.

It was during this short conversation that she answered my direct question and told me that Cathy could have a 90 to 95 percent chance of disease-free survival if we continued on the path that we started. I immediately noted that she conditioned her statistics, but wasn't sure what the conditions would be. She then explained that she was certain that the next phase of treatment would be chemotherapy using Adriamycin, which she characterized as a difficult but very effective drug.

I remember asking Alexandra when I could see Cathy. She told me that Dr. Disa was working on the reconstruction phase of the surgery, which would likely take another hour. Beyond that, she would be in the recovery room for a few hours. I asked Alexandra if she could be with me when I spoke to

Cathy because I so dreaded telling her about the spread to her lymph node. Cathy, however groggy, would understand the consequences of any nodal involvement, and she wasn't as foolishly optimistic as I was. Alexandra agreed to be with me when I explained the results, then added that she had to return to the operating room to prepare for the second of her five operations that day.

I was left feeling completely drained. I had expected that surgery would answer questions, and start us on a progression of good news after receiving only bad. Instead, it gave us more bad news and only created more questions. The principal questions we faced now were: 1) how far had the cancer spread, and 2) would the cancer be receptive to chemotherapy? We also needed to know if the cancer cells were estrogen receptor positive and Her2/Neu negative. These are important indicators of the likely efficacy of chemotherapy on cancer cells. We wouldn't know these answers until the pathology results came back a week later. The week promised to be grueling, not just because Cathy was post-op, but because if the pathology report came back bad it would have a profoundly negative impact on her progress.

I felt very letdown, but at least this time, I didn't have Phyllis on top of me. I had the luxury of sitting alone on that uncomfortable couch to piece together all that I'd just learned and determine how I would convey that information to our waiting friends and family. But because Phyllis had left me alone, I knew that I had an obligation to give her a fact-filled, straightforward recount of my discussion with Alexandra, and that I had to use the exact language that Alexandra used to allow Phyllis to draw her own inferences and make her own independent conclusions.

At that moment, I wanted to call my son Or in Israel. He always had the unique ability to be calm and strong no matter what was happening around him, as evidenced by his concern for me while he was lying in a hospital bed after his car accident. In fact, on the night of his accident, he demonstrated his ability to focus and stay calm as he crawled, while hurt, across the wet road and administered first aid to the injured occupants of the other car involved. There was a pay phone a few feet away and, for a second, I was really tempted to call him. But rather than dump my problems on my kid who just underwent his own surgery, I decided that I would emulate his sense of calm and strength when I went out to speak to my family and friends.

I did, however, put the pay phone to good use and called Jean Chin, Cathy's gynecologist, and told her what happened in the surgery. She was sympathetic and pretty blunt at the same time—she confirmed the same statistics that Alexandra had quoted me, then pointed out that there were some very recent studies, which showed little to no difference in the survival rates of women who had no nodal involvement and women who had some. She theorized that this might be attributed to the fact that women whose cancer is defined as Stage II cancer generally take chemotherapy, as opposed to Stage I, when patients often take no chemotherapy at all. She also told me about the recovery from the mastectomies and lymphadenectomy that Cathy had just undergone.

I sorted through what I learned from my short meeting with Dr. Heerdt and my phone conversation with Dr. Chin, then mentally made a list of what needed to be said:

● Cathy's disease-free survival chances could be as high as 95 percent if we do everything right going forward, which would involve much sacrifice of comfort.

● Cathy would undergo a rigorous course chemotherapy using Adriamycin, among other drugs.

• Cathy would be in severe physical pain for a week or two following the surgery.

• Cathy would certainly lose all of her hair during chemo.

• The pathology report from the breast tissue and lymph nodes that were taken from Cathy would provide significant information regarding her immediate and long-term future.

• We were still in for the fight of our lives and would have a pretty miserable year ahead. By no means did Cathy's surgery indicate that we were now out of the woods.

As I walked into the general waiting area to face Phyllis and our friends, nobody looked up at me or at least made eye contact. I noticed Rabbi Laine in the corner praying ferverently, and felt a collective sense of nervous anticipation from everyone. They respected that I might not have happy news and were giving me a little space and time to deal with all that was going on. I walked over to where my mom, Phyllis and Caryl were sitting and sat down next to my mother. Nobody crowded me for information, which allowed me a few seconds to get my bearings. I felt very safe sitting with my mom, as if she could make all of my problems go away like when I was a little boy. I was also comforted because at that moment I knew I had the love and concern of our friends in the waiting room, which was remarkably sustaining. I then patiently briefed our family and friends in factual, upbeat tones and suggested that it could be hours until Cathy woke up.

My mother very gracefully said nothing to me, yet her presence was reassuring. Aside from Cathy, she is the only other woman who has ever loved me completely. After a few seconds, I reassured Phyllis that Cathy's chances of surviving today were 100 percent and as high as 95 percent regarding long-term, disease-free survival. I stressed to Phyllis that this was Dr. Heerdt's take, not mine. I figured I had time to tell them about the chemotherapy part later. After all, it was her daughter and she was having trouble grasping all that was happening to Cathy, so she gained a sense of calm from mine.

Our friends started to surround me with love and support, and the positive energy I particularly felt from Cathy's closest girlfriends fortified me for the long road ahead. Everybody there quickly digested that we still had much to do to beat this cancer. This whole thing was tough on Cathy's closest girlfriend Caryl, but she threw her support around me, knowing that this is what Cathy wanted her to do. I pulled Caryl aside and asked her to take care of Phyllis, to ease her pain and stress, since Phyllis really had nobody there for her. Caryl handled this tough task, which made waiting for Cathy to come out of the anesthesia a bit easier for me. She was worried about her dearest friend, but was charged with watching out for me by Cathy's wishes, and Phyllis by mine—her plate was pretty full.

Soon Dr. Disa appeared and informed me that the reconstructive aspect of today's surgery went very well. I remember hearing that Dr. Heerdt left me with lots of skin to work with." My concern was more with Cathy's health and less with the reconstruction. I didn't fully understand at that point how important the latter would be to Cathy's psychological well being.

Within a few hours, I was able to see Cathy in the recovery room. She was so affected by the anesthesia that she stayed asleep longer than anyone would have guessed. Alexandra had already left and I was alone to break the news to her. As she stirred in her bed, I held her hand and told her that the cancer went to her sentinel node, but that it didn't appear to have spread farther. Cathy, without opening her eyes said, "I know, Alexandra already spoke to me. I know it spread but also know that it will be all right." I was extremely relieved that Cathy knew and accepted this so bravely. It was identical to her reaction when I told her three weeks earlier that we would need to have both breasts removed. Her ability to deal with adversity was quite remarkable. Courage is the ability to face the unknown, and Cathy was demonstrating great courage.

As I sat next to her in the recovery room. I noticed the drains coming out of her body from just under her armpits. This is common practice after a mastectomy, in which the surgeon inserts tubes through the skin into the armpit with a clear plastic ball at the end. It's designed to be airtight and provide a modest amount of suction into the newly created surgically formed cavity where the fluid accumulates, permitting the skin to adhere to the pectoralis muscle so that there are no air lumps on the breast mound. These drains stay in a patient for about ten days, or until the body stops creating excess fluid. It is a bit of an ordeal emptying the drains while not disturbing the tubes themselves, but the nurses teach you how and you just do it. While Cathy was lying on her bed, I also noted that her breast mounds were significantly smaller than they were just a few hours earlier. She still had mounds but they were not pronounced at all. All in all, my wife looked pretty beat up.

Cathy had considerable difficulty shaking off the effects of the anesthesia. Before surgery, we were really clueless about anesthesia, and considered it and its administration to be easily commoditized. Anesthesia, however, isn't a commodity at all, and is actually composed of two parts. The first part makes a patient sleep, while the second part—the narcotic—is used to block the pain receptors. Together, they put a patient to sleep and prevent them from waking up in screaming agony during surgery. Unfortunately, the narcotic portion of the anesthesia makes some patients—especially highly allergic people like Cathy—very nauseous. It is interesting that we interviewed surgeons and spent time learning about many of the challenges and issues that Cathy would face relative to her cancer, yet we didn't even think to consider any aspects of anesthesiology, notwithstanding our knowledge that Cathy was allergic to many narcotic—type substances. Cathy's system, for whatever reason, just couldn't handle the aftereffects of the narcotic. While in the recovery room, she was overcome with nausea and retched violently, but couldn't vomit as her system was empty. The retching caused great discomfort because her body, while still largely numb, had undergone such an invasive surgical procedure. All we could do was ask the recovery nurses for more Kytril or Zofran. What we learned a little too late is that if you ask for an antiemetic (anti-nausea medication) after nausea has set in, it is too late for it to be effective. We would soon learn the same thing about pain medication. *Anticipation* of nausea and pain is the key to their management.

By 1:00 P.M., Cathy was still too sick to leave the recovery room, so I asked her friends to leave as she was likely going to be in there for a few more hours. I promised everyone that I would brief them via email that night. I had already prepared an email distribution list of about fifty concerned family members and friends that I would keep informed of Cathy's condition. Just after 3:00 P.M., we were able to take Cathy to her room. While she was very uncomfortable, she showed some signs that the nausea was fading. I arranged for a private room, feeling that 135 square feet to ourselves would ease the discomfort in the hours and days that lay ahead.

I spent as much time as possible that afternoon with Cathy, but was mindful that my two boys at home were very concerned about their mom and needed my loving reassurance. I asked my parents to leave the hospital and spend time with their grandkids while I stayed a few more hours at the hospital with Cathy. At about 7:30 P.M. as Cathy slept, I went into a small lounge on the tenth floor, where I used one of two computers there to access my computer at work and my prearranged email distribution list of friends and family. I then sent the following email:

Surgery — It's Not An Amputation

Wednesday, January 08, 2003

I am writing this from Memorial Sloan-Kettering Cancer Center.
Today has been and still is a very long and tough day with generally good results.
Cathy's surgery was successful. She is resting (actually sleeping) after approximately four hours of surgery, which began at 7:30 this morning.

We are deeply appreciative of all of the expressions of support that we received. During her surgery, surrounded by friends and family, I felt like we had a home team advantage.

*The coming weeks and months promise to be grueling...but that is okay because we are completely focused on beating this cancer. We believe that the cancer was removed surgically today, but **both** understand that the next steps, which will include aggressive chemotherapy, will test us. I know my beautiful and courageous wife will continue to inspire all of us with the way she faces chemotherapy, and any and all other challenges that lie ahead.*

In addition to being a kind and giving person, Cathy is tough as nails, and I am very proud of her.

Mark

I knew that I didn't want to make fifty phone calls. The email seemed to work, as mostly everyone on the distribution list responded and thanked me for letting them know what was happening.

Before leaving for the evening, I met many of the nurses on the floor, and was amazed by their sense of compassion for their patients and their dexterity in handling the postoperative women on the floor. Cathy was in pain, nauseous and had tubes coming out of her body, yet the nurses navigated around her body professionally, almost effortlessly. Their touch caused Cathy no discomfort.

Cathy's room was on the tenth floor of MSKCC, which was only for women with breast and ovarian cancers. There were women recovering from a broad range of procedures, from lumpectomies, mastectomies and oophorectomies to women who were in their last few days of life, about to succumb to ovarian cancer. The woman in the room right next to Cathy's was about to die after a long battle with ovarian cancer. Her quiet sobs and occasional shrill cries of "Lord take me, I'm ready," sliced to my core. I was grateful that Cathy was in a place that understood how to deal with her pain and discomfort, but knew that she wouldn't heal until she was in her own bed. Despite the staff's attempts to create a soothing environment, the tenth floor was loud and chaotic and there were echoes of pain and suffering down every hallway.

The nurses on the floor were genuinely nice people and I got along well with them. They must have realized how I marveled at their dexterity and professionalism as I carefully observed their movements, determined to learn as much as I possibly could about caring for Cathy.

The team of social workers on the tenth floor was also wonderful. They were there to support the nursing staff, the physicians, and the families of the patients as well as the patients themselves. The social workers helped me deal with Cathy's mom and with my own children. They were also pretty terrific in dealing with me. I thought I was on good behavior, but there were days that I seemed to just look for reasons to argue with Phyllis (and Phyllis gave me plenty of reasons), and other days when I was absolutely obsessive about cleaning Cathy's room.

In the days following Cathy's surgery, she was in a constant state of discomfort. To make matters worse, the tubes and monitors attached to her arms limited her movement; she was unable to adjust her positioning and ease her pain. The only ones who could adjust her were the nurses, but they couldn't be by her side constantly. On the third day after her surgery, Cathy was particularly uncomfortable because she was trying to reduce her intake of pain medication (morphine). She asked me to help her sit up slightly in her bed. I stepped forward and did exactly what I'd watched the nurses do several times: I put my left hand directly under her, between her shoulder blades. I put her hands on my shoulders so that in one coordinated move, Cathy could lift herself off the bed using my shoulders as leverage, while my hand provided an even and steady lift for her upper torso.

It seemed simple enough when I watched the nurses do it, but this time something went wrong. I didn't fully anticipate that Cathy's hands around my shoulders would be as weak as they were, and inadvertently applied a bit too much pressure between her shoulder blades. Instead of wincing in pain, Cathy shrieked in agony and began to cry loudly. Phyllis, coincidentally, walked into the room when the incident occurred, and we looked at each other helplessly, realizing that neither of us could do anything for Cathy at that point.

I ran out of the room to the nurses' station and told them, "I just hurt my wife and think I may have opened her surgical wounds while trying to lift her." The nurses immediately ran into the room, while I moved myself into the corner and focused on not interfering as they checked to see what damage I had caused my crying wife. The nurses moved quickly to find the source of the injury as they were concerned by the way I described what happened and because Cathy was crying in such searing pain.

I watched as the nurses quickly stripped off Cathy's gown, exposing her post surgical breasts, while Cathy heaved in paroxysms of pain—pain that I had caused. I wanted nothing more than to help or comfort my wife, but I couldn't be of any use whatsoever in that situation. I slumped to the floor and cried a helpless, sleep-deprived, emotionally overwrought cry, convinced that I had carelessly injured my wife. Furthermore, I had envisioned seeing Cathy's post surgical breasts when she was ready to show them to me. This wasn't the way it was supposed to go. I was mortified because not only did I hurt my wife, but I also humiliated her by having her breasts exposed to her mother and me before she was able to even look tat hem herself. Cathy was in horrific pain, stripped of her femininity and dignity because I mistimed "my lift" and overestimated my ability to help. My sadness and pain at that moment had reached a new low.

After Cathy was stabilized, we spoke to the nurses and the on-duty surgical resident about what had happened. As it was explained, I really hadn't mishandled Cathy all that badly. The fact that her morphine was wearing off, combined with her exhaustion and emotionally shattered postoperative state, largely contributed to the incident. The lift caused a "tug" on her drains, which in turn unleashed a waterfall of emotion that she couldn't control. The nurses referred to the tug as a "zinger." Notwithstanding the mild term the nurses used, I was afraid to touch Cathy after that event for no less than a month.

That night, when I arrived home from the hospital, Brandon and Ryan were asleep in my bed, which was not uncommon. Instead of carrying them to their beds, I got into my bed next to them and held them while I fell into a dreamless, black sleep of pure emotional and physical exhaustion. The next morning I awoke tired and still drained from the emotions of the previous night. If my defense mechanism of denial had been telling me that getting through this wouldn't be a difficult ordeal, that notion was completely erased, as it was apparent that I would have no shortcuts or hiding places available to me.

I had always believed that expressions like "one step at a time" and "one day at a time" were ridiculous and didn't apply to me. Suddenly, they had tremendous application to how and what I was feeling. I realized that each day would present new challenges, and that, I couldn't afford to expend much energy on tomorrow until I was comfortable that I was through today. My expectations of myself as a supportive husband had fallen precipitously in the past twenty-four hours. I faced the fact that I wasn't Superman, but just a regular guy who was going to make many of the mistakes regular men make when supporting a sick wife. This shattered my confidence because I was so focused on being Superman and holding it together for Cathy.

On a sunny Sunday morning, only five days after her surgery, I brought Cathy home from the hospital. It was bittersweet because it relieved the boys of so much stress, yet it created another type of stress—Cathy was still feeling and looking miserable. Our doormen had a look of horror when they saw her come out of the car and into our building with such a pained and slow gait. I had gently warned our sons that they could kiss, but not hug Mommy, because she was sore from her surgery. They complied and instinctively understood how to be gentle with their mother. The relief on their faces and the comfort of being in her own bed was a great tonic for her.

During her first days home, Cathy needed my help going to the bathroom and washing herself. I was glad to be finally able to help my wife and found no task too personal. I wanted to be as attentive as I could because I knew that she would have been as attentive to me if the situations were somehow reversed. I also believe that by nursing Cathy back to health, I was able to regain a modicum of control, and that aided in my healing. At night, I slept on an air mattress that I put on the floor next to our bed. At first, I told myself that I wanted to do this so that I could be right beneath Cathy and immediately responsive to her moaning or turning in bed. In reality, I was afraid to share a bed with her in case I would move in my sleep and inadvertently "tug" on her drains. I was scared to hurt my wife again with another zinger because this time, there wouldn't be any nurses around to bail me out.

By the time Cathy was released from the hospital, she had a good understanding of how to administer pain medication, and a greater knowledge of what would and wouldn't work for her. Percoset didn't work at all; it just made her nauseous. Dilaudid apparently worked pretty well, but needed to be taken before the pain started. Together we learned that pain management is really just pain anticipation, and once pain has started, it's very hard to treat. Furthermore, as pain begins, patients tend to tense up waiting for the medication to kick in, which in turn causes tension that increases the pain and diminishes the effect of the medication.

Cathy voiced concern to me about the addictive qualities of certain pain medication—especially Dilaudid, since it is opium based and not only relieved the pain, but also literally got her high. I heard her, but didn't really listen because I wanted so badly to alleviate her constant discomfort.

As Cathy became more experienced with anticipating and dealing with her postoperative pain, we were somewhat relieved but also concerned that she could become addicted to pain medication. At most hospitals, this is a real concern, but at most cancer centers, there is less concern about addiction and more focus on survival. The general but unspoken wisdom at cancer hospitals is that they will deal with addiction later. However, as we discovered, this is not always the case.

After surgery there is a lag of about a month before chemotherapy begins (provided it is even necessary). During the first part of this month, the patient is in the hospital, where morphine can be self-administered by a PCA, a device that allows patients to inject a modest amount of morphine directly into their IVs. Once a patient comes off morphine, but is still in the hospital, oral pain medication can be administered only by a nurse.

The lag times between calling a nurse and receiving the pain medication often misses the window of time when the pain can be successfully ameliorated. Missing this window causes anxiety, which of course keeps the patient awake at night, and thereby, retards healing, because restful sleep is essential to recovery.

By the time the patient arrives home with a bottle full of painkillers, they have been moderately traumatized by the fear of pain as much as the pain itself. Cancer centers often do not have the services and support systems necessary, especially on an outpatient basis, to wean patients off addictive medications. The patient and her family are often left to their own devices to deal with any resulting addictions.

CHAPTER 5

CHEMOTHERAPY—HOW TO DEAL WITH THE CHEMO SHARK

Chemotherapy is a necessary evil. While many times it can eradicate cancer within a person's body, it wreaks havoc, both short-term and long-term, on that same body. There are two basic types of chemotherapy (chemo); adjuvant chemotherapy and neoadjuvant chemotherapy. Most women being treated for breast cancer are given adjuvant chemotherapy, which is "just in case" therapy in that it is given after surgery in the event that undetectable, microscopic cancer cells that weren't eliminated surgically are insidiously multiplying inside the woman's body. While traditional breast surgery typically rids the body of the detectable and visible cancer cells, chemo attacks and presumably kills whatever may be left. After appropriate surgery for breast cancer, there can be up to a 75 percent chance (assuming there was early detection and competent surgical and/or radiological intervention) that all cancer cells were removed. Adjuvant chemotherapy wouldn't be necessary if there was a test available that could detect the presence of microscopic traces of cancer. Since no such test presently exists, many physicians feel it is advisable to act as if surgery was only able to eliminate the visible cancer cells. I agree with this way of thinking, and so does Cathy.

Neoadjuvant chemotherapy is an important life-saving tool because it is given before surgery to shrink or even eliminate a patient's tumors, and enhance the surgeon's chances for success. Several leading cancer hospitals are now utilizing neoadjuvant chemotherapy to effectively rid the patient of cancer cells, which can lessen the need for very invasive or extreme surgery. Until recently, neoadjuvant chemotherapy was given only to cancer patients with tumors or lesions that were in a place or of a size that made surgery unfeasible. Either way, adjuvant and neoadjuvant chemotherapy are important and potent weapons in the fight against many different cancers, especially breast cancer.

Unfortunately, chemo takes a toll on those who take it and those who care for them. While Cathy suffered through chemotherapy, we all suffered as we watched and felt her vitality and energy being steadily drained. In addition to losing her stamina, we had to stand by and watch her lose her hair, her appetite and her normally glowing, healthful pallor. Cathy's greatest frustration during chemotherapy was living at home with her family, but not being able to do the things for her family that she was accustomed to doing, and that we were accustomed to having her do. Her debilitation caused her grievous emotional pain because of the profound effects of worry and stress for Brandon and Ryan.

In processing the concept that there was a 75 percent chance that chemo was unnecessary and could have lifelong negative health consequences, I needed to understand its potential benefits as well as Cathy's prescribed protocol was designed to do and what side effects might come with it. Understanding the process and the nature of the drugs she would take made living through the very rough four months of treatment somehow more manageable, perhaps because I allowed myself to think that a little knowledge was also a little control. It also allowed me to visualize how these toxic agents, which were turning Cathy's world upside-down, were actually attacking hidden cancer cells.

Cathy's protocol consisted of three drugs: Adriamycin, Cytoxan and Taxol. These drugs were administered every two weeks for a period of four months. The first four sessions, which consisted of IV drips of Adriamycin and Cytoxan, were terrible. By comparison, the last four sessions, which consisted of 6-hour infusions of Taxol, were not nearly as bad. The drugs affected Cathy both positively and negatively in different ways. Many women have different experiences with these drugs, as some are lightly affected by Adriamycin and Cytoxan but debilitated by Taxol. The opposite was true with Cathy—she was debilitated by Adriamycin and Cytoxan, but not terribly impacted by Taxol. Taxol bloats most women and they suffer significant weight gain, but it never bloated Cathy. My point, which is reinforced by anyone who is knowledgeable about chemotherapy, is that there is no practical way to predict the side effects of these drugs on any individual woman, since all women react differently to them.

Chemotherapy drugs work in five different ways. Vinca alkaloids inhibit cancer cells' ability to multiply, antimetoblites (like Methotrexate) starve the cancer cells while they are multiplying, and anti-tumor antibiotics slow the growth of the cancer cells. Alkylating agents like Cytoxan and Adriamycin, bind with the cancer cells so that they lose their ability to divide, and natural products like Taxol, which is made from the Pacific yew tree, interferes with the basic cellular architecture and division of the cancer cells. If these different agents had the ability to attack cancer cells only and stop them from multiplying, starve them, slow their growth, latch healthy cells to them so they couldn't divide, and alter their basic architecture, then the cancer patient would endure chemotherapy easily. Unfortunately, these agents aren't completely accurate when attacking cancer cells, and they sometimes attack perfectly healthy cells. This attack of healthy cells is what creates the side effects that everyone has heard about and which can be quite profound. Sometimes they are severe enough to permanently damage the patient's heart, lungs or other vital organs. The difficult part of gauging this damage is that doctors generally cannot tell who will respond well and who will be damaged by the treatment. This is why they assess a patient's age and overall health as well as the type of cancer they are treating when prescribing a chemotherapy regimen.

When chemotherapy agents begin attacking tumors, they also attack the host (the body). Unfortunately, the body, sensing this invasion of attacking agents, mounts its own fight against them. Generally, it is a losing and exhausting fight as the chemotherapy agents deplete the body's immune system by adversely affecting the patient's bone marrow, where the white blood cells that fight infection are produced. In order to restore the production of white blood cells, many chemotherapy patients are prescribed a colony—stimulating factor called Neupogen. This medication, which is administered with nightly injections between chemo cycles, will build up a patient's immune system and provide the patient with the ability—if they and their oncologist choose—to take chemotherapy every two weeks instead of every three weeks. Without Neupogen, Cathy's immune system would not have been able to adequately withstand taking chemo every two weeks. This "high-density dosing" enhances chemo's effectiveness and allows a patient to finish treatment in four months rather than six. The downside is that the patient feels pretty awful for the entire four months, as opposed to feeling awful for only 66 percent of the time over six months.

The theory on taking chemotherapy every two weeks instead of every three is both simple and somewhat elegant. Each chemotherapy session could kill 90 percent of any cancer cells in the body that were not eliminated through surgery. The remaining 10 percent of hidden cancer cells that survived the onslaught of the chemotherapy agents will start to multiply almost immediately after each session. Rather than allow the surviving cells to multiply for three weeks, they get reduced again by 90 percent within two weeks before their multiplication has taken hold. The cells multiply by dividing, which makes the consequence of interdicting the cell multiplication two-thirds into their growth pattern twice as effective as waiting for the full three weeks. By the time the patient has undergone eight sessions in rapid sequence, there is a statistically insignificant amount of cancer cells in the body. Cathy used Neupogen injections, which I administered at home, to take chemotherapy every two weeks.

During this process, I learned that different hospitals and doctors have different views on chemotherapy, and that it is not a process that can be looked at as a commodity. The intense patient monitoring and frequent adjustments make the administration of chemotherapy an interactive science as well as an art. In order to minimize complications from the chemo drugs and maximize their effectiveness, physicians, nurses and patients need to take into consideration a patient's goals, their overall health, and the support systems available to the patient.

For the Weiss family, there was no question that we wanted to attack Cathy's cancer with whatever chemotherapy resources were available. We were also quite intrepid about the side effects of these resources; Cathy was in excellent health before her surgery, and she was prepared to make any sacrifice that would enhance the likelihood of living to raise her two boys and grow old with me. Many women, however, don't have young children or are at a stage in life where the corrosive effects of chemotherapy may compromise other vital aspects of their health to the point that the cure might be worse than the risk of their cancer's recurrence. Additionally, many women who are confronted with these different options don't have the support system of family and friends, or the financial wherewithal to allow them to stand up to the rigors of chemo.

Two weeks after Cathy's surgery, Dr. Heerdt reviewed her positive pathology report with us. We were fortunate because Cathy's tumor was Her2/Neu negative and estrogen receptor positive. This meant that there was a high probability that Cathy would respond to a standard regimen of chemotherapy.

Besides giving us some good news at this appointment, Dr. Heerdt recommended an oncologist at MSKCC named Chau Dang. Chau is a brilliant young woman who is accessible, caring, conscientious and a very effective communicator whose responsiveness was not limited exclusively to Cathy. She answered all of my questions in meticulous detail, and may have been mildly amused by how much basic information I ingested in a short amount of time. Because Chau quickly and decisively earned our trust and confidence, there was no question that for the foreseeable future, she was going to quarterback Cathy's healthcare.

Many patients and their families think they will find some sort of treatment edge on the Internet, which is unknown to their oncologist. This is both ridiculous and unlikely if the patient is being treated at an established cancer center or a respected teaching hospital. At MSKCC, the oncologists who treat breast cancer patients work in a collaborative environment under the leadership of renowned oncologist Larry Norton. Dr. Norton and his team, which includes Dr. Dang, develop the chemotherapy protocols for all of MSKCC's breast cancer patients based on the staging of each patient's cancer. The entire team has tremendous access to cutting-edge information and research so that their collaborative approach insures that all patients receive the collective experience of the oncology department at MSKCC and beyond

Notwithstanding the confidence we had in Dr. Norton's department, I was more fearful of chemotherapy than I was of surgery, largely because surgery was of shorter duration and more predictable in how it would impact Cathy. There are some women who take rigorous courses of chemotherapy and have little to no side effects, and others who take mild courses and suffer greatly.

Cathy took a rigorous course and suffered terribly; she was very sensitive to all of the meds that were administered. Her chemo started in early February and was immediately tough on her. Three days after her first treatment, when we expected some relief from the headaches and nausea,

I woke up around 5 A.M. to the sound of a thud—Cathy fell out of bed. I got up and went to pick her up as she was crawling on the floor toward the bathroom. She was crying and moaning that she needed to vomit but couldn't, as she hadn't eaten anything solid in a few days. Her pale, sweaty body was gripped in pain from the top of her head to right behind her eyes and all the way down to her stomach.

I helped her to the bathroom and held her as she wretched unproductively. Unfortunately, the sounds of Cathy's retching as well as the commotion coming from our room woke up Brandon and Ryan. They came into our room together in their pajamas while rubbing sleep from their eyes to see what was happening. I almost dropped Cathy as I ran to block them from coming into the bathroom and seeing their mother in such sorry shape. I hustled them to the den on the far side of our apartment, then ran back to find Cathy on the bathroom floor, asleep in a puddle of greenish clear liquid that she managed to throw up. I cleaned her up and carried her back to bed, then quickly cleaned the bathroom floor. I spent the next two hours calming, feeding and getting my kids ready for school while comforting and cleaning Cathy as she tried several more times to make it to the bathroom to vomit. At the same time I called Maureen, the boys' babysitter, at home and asked her to come to our house earlier than usual to help me.

None of what had happened here made sense; it was Day 4 after chemo and Cathy was supposed to be feeling better than she had in Days 1 through 3. All the while, I was emailing Chau, trying to find out what was happening and how to make it stop. Emails went directly to Chau's pager whereas leaving a message at the hospital was pointless, since whatever operator took the call would simply email her and ask her to call us. Chau had told me when we first met that email-to-email would accelerate response time. I kept telling Cathy that Chau would call at any moment, while I considered calling an ambulance to take her to the hospital. I wondered if this was a serious problem or a predictable side effect of the treatments. And if it was a predictable side effect, why wasn't I told that there could be days this bad, or that Day 4 could be significantly worse than Day 3?

I finally got Brandon onto his bus—which was a half-hour late because of a huge traffic jam in Manhattan caused by President Bush's motorcade (he was in New York to address the United Nations and prevail upon the world that Iraq possessed weapons of mass destruction)—just as Maureen came. I told her that I would take Ryan to school, so she need-ed to stay with Cathy and have the phone nearby as I was expecting an important call from our oncologist. If Chau hadn't called by the time I took Ryan to school, I would take Cathy to MSKCC's version of an emergency room. I showered, changed into a gray flannel suit and was about to leave, but by then Ryan knew something was very wrong and refused to get into his stroller.

On the rare days that I was able to take him to nursery school before Cathy got sick, we would talk and laugh during our twenty-minute walk. This day however, he immediately started to cry as soon as we left our front door. He complained loudly through his tears that he "hated every-one and everything." For the next twenty minutes, my focus was split between cheering up my son, waiting for my cell phone to ring, and con-stantly checking my Blackberry for an email response from Chau. I started singing funny songs to Ryan as we walked. After a while, I carried him on my shoulders part of the way, walked backwards with him in the stroller, and pretended that he was me and I was him. As I put all of my effort into insulating Ryan from our trouble at home I felt a bit like Roberto Benini in Life is Beautiful. It took about fifteen minutes and considerable effort before he laughed and became my happy three-year-old once more. As I dropped Ryan off at school, I saw all of these happy, loving parents and felt a surge of bitterness that they were focusing on play dates and dinner parties while my plate was full with Cathy's medical problems. Then, four minutes after I dropped off Ryan, Chau called me on my cell phone. She said that she had spoken to Cathy and advised her to take something that would chemically balance her and provide instant relief. When I called home and heard Cathy's voice, I knew right away that she felt much better.

The cause of Cathy's misery was the rapid reduction of the combination of Zofran, Dilaudid and Valium that she was taking. The Zofran was used for the nausea, the Valium was used to palliate her constant headaches caused by the Zofran, and the Dilaudid is the highly addictive pain medication that Cathy was still taking, partly for the headaches from the chemo and partly because she still had some pain from the surgery. Cathy had experienced classic withdrawal from all of the meds we used to alleviate the effects of surgery as well as the Adriamycin and Cytoxan. She had simply reduced these medications too quickly and had no idea of the intense reaction she would suffer. Finding the right combination of meds that counteract the effects of chemo is a vicious art form that is usually accomplished successfully, but with a moderate amount of trial and error. In our case, though, the amount of trial and error appeared to be more than moderate.

I remember finishing the phone calls with Chau and Cathy and then looking at my reflection in a storefront window at 64th Street and Madison Avenue. I saw a tired and beaten man completely drained of vitality, and I still had to go to work and prepare for a significant new business presentation that afternoon. I went home twice that day for quick visits and surprisingly did a credible job in my afternoon presentation. I finished my other business then went home to take care of the children and Cathy. That night, after everyone was asleep, I worked for an hour or so; I found that I was so wound up by the events of the day, and by how far behind I was at work, that my mind literally raced from topic to topic. When I finally went to bed, I was feeling exhausted, but it still took me awhile to fall asleep. I ultimately faded off, hoping that tomorrow would be easier.

While the "withdrawal day" was certainly taxing on all of us, twelve days later Cathy and I had another experience that was every bit as emotionally grueling. Many women know this as the day they lost their hair. Two days into the second chemo cycle, Cathy called me at work and said that her scalp was tingling and that hair was falling out in clumps. She then emailed me an hour later to let me know that she was going to "Willie's," the woman who cuts both our hair—and was going to ask her to shave her head. Cathy already had a series of severe haircuts that had reduced her long blond hair to stylish but very short. The progressively shorter haircuts were designed to allow her and our kids the ability to accept that her long blonde hair would soon be gone. Common wisdom suggests that it is better psychologically for a woman to have her head shaved rather than let her hair fall out over the course of a few days.

When I saw this email, I ran out of my office and got home just in time to intercept Cathy. I told her I'd get Willie to come to our house and do it. We both like and trust Willie and know all the people who work in her salon, but the idea of being in a hair salon and letting other clients—complete strangers—watch Cathy's head get shaved was just too painful to even think about. Ordinarily, women get their heads shaved in the wig salon, but Cathy hadn't done this yet because she unreasonably hoped that somehow her hair wouldn't fall out. And now, on the day that her hair started to fall out in large clumps, the wig salon was closed!

I ran to Willie's, which is only one block from our apartment and told her what was going on. She dropped what she was doing and came to our house with whatever tools she needed. I held my wife's hand as Willie shaved Cathy's beautiful blonde hair in our kitchen. Liz, who works for us, periodically helping at home, was also in the room, and she grabbed a dustpan and broom to clean up Cathy's beautiful hair while it was still being shaved off. I considered this to be such a deeply personal act that I took the dustpan and broom from Liz and cleaned up Cathy's hair myself. I'm not sure why, but I felt it was appropriate for me to participate in this painful ritual.

Cathy was being brave, but crying nonetheless. Losing her beautiful breasts and her lustrous hair within five weeks was hard to handle; she had been stripped of two elements of her femininity in a condensed period of time. Part of the difficulty, undoubtedly, was that while her hair was gone, it wasn't even going to start growing back for four or five months. We were just at the beginning of chemotherapy, and had what felt like a very long road ahead of us.

The hardest part for me that morning was being unable to help comfort my wife during such a traumatic time. She lost her hair, which she had been dreading since she woke up from surgery, and it was truly as horrible as she had anticipated. I am thankful that I had the presence of mind not to say anything to try to make her feel better, as it would have rung hollow. A comment like, "It will grow back," wouldn't have done her any good because intellectually, she already knew this. She just needed time to process it. I held and kissed her, and whispered that I loved her and would always be there for her. This was the right—and probably only—thing for me to say.

Cathy wrapped herself in a quilt and sat on the couch. She asked me to go back to work and assured me that she would be fine. It was a hollow assurance, but Cathy needed to process this miserable event and felt that she could best do it without watching me suffer through it with her. She was pale, gaunt and now bald, but her eyes still held the look of a brave and determined fighter who had plenty of fight in her.

I went back to the office, but was only there physically. Mentally, I was a million miles away. It was hard to think about real estate when I was just sweeping all of my wife's hair into a dustpan. I tried to maintain my bearings and resolve to hold it all together, even though I knew that the real pain of chemotherapy would be not just days like this, but the long-term emotional toll it would take on all of us. I felt that living through this with Cathy and the boys was taking the last few remnants of my youth, as I knew the word "carefree" would never be applicable to my life again. Looking back to that day, I think I mourned the loss of my youth. I was now in midlife no matter how I looked or felt—and I wasn't looking or feeling very young.

Many women hope against hope that they won't lose their hair, but with toxic agents like Adriamycin, a woman's hair is actually doomed to fall out as soon as she takes the first treatment. Adriamycin kills the hair at the root, though doesn't cause it to fall out on the spot because while the root is killed, the scalp holds the individual strands of hair in place. Two weeks later, immediately before the next treatment, as a new root starts to grow, it forces the dead roots from the scalp, which causes the hair to fall out in clumps. The new root gets killed the same way in a miserable cycle of baldness that doesn't end until two weeks after chemotherapy treatments end.

Chemotherapy drugs are cumulative in a person's system, which generally means that the treatments are worse each time. Conversely, once the treatments are over, it takes some time for the drugs to actually leave the patient's system. During chemo however, patients learn how to mitigate its cumulative effects with increased knowledge of their own drug sensitivities and increased knowledge on how to successfully counteract the meds. In short, chemo gets progressively worse, but you get better at dealing with it.

Fortunately for Cathy, the first four sessions were significantly worse than the last four as Adriamycin and Cytoxan were much harder on her system than Taxol. However, at the time of this writing, Cathy is suffering from some mild arthritis in her hands, which the doctors think is a result of the treatment with Taxol. I've heard from other women that while Adriamycin and Cytoxan weren't so bad, Taxol had caused all kinds of problems like bloating and weight gain as well as physical pain. I now understand why, before Cathy started chemo, no woman we spoke to who had gone through it would tell us too much about her experiences. They knew that chemotherapy could be tough or easy, and that there is no rational way to anticipate any individual's reaction. Nobody wanted to minimize a harrowing process or overstate what could be a mild experience for others.

Pretty much all of the women with whom we spoke advised us to be very careful with diet to read about the do's and don'ts during chemotherapy. Ice chips during the treatments were in, though foods with acid were out! The oncologist offered guidelines that were important to follow, and we also listened to insights from the chemotherapy nurses.

Cathy found that exercise actually helped her metabolize the chemo drugs; it helped them to not only work, but to get out of her system faster. Our friends, Richard and Amy Miller own a business called the Gym Source and were gracious enough to lend us a really nice recumbent bicycle that we kept in our bedroom. Cathy tried to spend some time each day on the bike and was generally able to make it. Of course, there were days when she couldn't ride it at all, or only stay on it for a minute or two... but there were other days when she was actually able to ride for thirty minutes. This moderate amount of exercise gave Cathy a little more control of her body and made the process of regaining control of her body and life after chemotherapy ended much easier. A recumbent bike worked because it put little to no strain or jarring on Cathy's surgically traumatized upper body. Many women use yoga for the same purpose. Whether its biking, yoga or a gentle walk, I am a big proponent of exercise during treatment. It is one small way for a woman to expedite feeling like herself again.

During the four months of chemotherapy, we grew accustomed to the cyclicality of life revolving around "chemo day." Invariably, chemo day was followed by about a week of Cathy feeling really bad. We called these periods "chemo weeks" and learned not to schedule anything of consequence during them, as Cathy's general level of strength and overall morale would be low. Her chemo was always on a Tuesday, and for the duration of the process our friends, Judy Hundley and Marc Cummings, sent us a spectacular meal from the kitchen of their catering company, Gracious Thyme. Cathy was usually too nauseous to eat, but the boys and I looked forward to those well-balanced, delicious meals.

More of the days during the following week—the non-chemo week— would be significantly better, and Cathy would busy herself doing all of the things that she couldn't do the previous week. The weekend before treatments usually started out really well because they were the most distant days from the last treatment. However, on those Sunday nights the sense of anxiety that the treatment was about to start all over again became pervasive. This became our pattern and we actually got used to it. The first four sessions produced more anxiety than the last four not just because Adriamycin was more difficult than Taxol, but because we started to sense that we were getting close to the end of Cathy's treatments. Each day that passed during chemo became a day closer to the end of it. I imagine prison inmates feel the same way.

The entire chemotherapy experience rests in my memory as a dark passage of unpleasantness. The only bright spot was on May 9 at 2:34 P.M., when Cathy called me from her cell phone as she and her friends Jill, Janie and Leslie were leaving MSKCC. I was walking in a light drizzle, crossing Lexington Avenue at 55th Street on my way to meet her at the hospital, when I answered my cell and heard her say, "Mark, I love you... We just finished." Our chemotherapy ordeal had finally ended. After a momentary feeling of numbness, I got an endorphin high, as if I ran ten miles fast. Only this high grew and grew, and lasted a full month. For us, finishing chemo was a wonderful milestone in our fight against breast cancer, as we both knew that the most grueling part of Cathy's treatment was behind us. We were also naãve enough to think that from that point on, recovery and adapting back into our normal lives would be relatively easy. We hadn't yet grasped the long-term physical and emotional consequences of treatment for breast cancer.

Two weeks after Cathy's last chemotherapy session, I remember being in a fabulous mood. I called my mom in Florida and told her that I was having the best Tuesday of my life—not only was Cathy not in that chemo chair with an IV in her arm, but we also started to notice that her hair was growing back. During the previous four months, it would always start to grow back toward the end of a cycle, only to be knocked out by the next round of chemo. This time, we knew it would come back and keep on coming. I felt true relief because I knew that healing, both physical and emotional, had begun in earnest.

Two weeks later, or a month after chemo ended, Cathy and I took a mini-jog to Central Park. Before Cathy got sick, we would sometimes run the few blocks from our apartment on 79th Street to the park and then a few miles in the park—usually around the Jacquelyn Kennedy Onassis Reservoir. That beautiful June morning, we jogged to the park and halfway home for a total of a mile, which was triumphant in every way. Cathy was exhilarated when we returned home, so much so that she started running everyday and gradually built up her mileage. The more she ran, the faster her body rid itself of the toxins that coursed through her veins for the last sixteen weeks. As the toxins dissipated, she felt better, and the better she felt, the more she wanted to run. The more she ran, the better she looked, and the better she looked, the better she felt. This incredible productive cycle was only limited by our concern that she not push herself too hard and get injured. Ironically, Lance Armstrong shattered this concern—it was around this time that he was staging his dramatic comeback, and on his way to winning his fifth consecutive Tour de France.

Cathy had been running about a mile and a half every day until that day in late June, when Lance received the yellow jersey for being the leader. His picture the next morning was on the front pages of *The New York Times* and *New York Post*. That morning Cathy ran three miles, went home and picked up our new puppy Sami, then took her for a long walk. She called me exhausted and exhilarated because Lance Armstrong's inspiring comeback in the Tour De France gave her the confidence to push herself as hard as she could. By late July, Cathy was running five miles every morning, and would also take long bike rides most afternoons.

Cathy and the boys spent the entire summer at our house in Westhampton Beach. I commuted to see them on weekends and was able to take the last three weeks of the summer off for a much—needed vacation. I was able to surround my family with love and warmth, which was great for all of us. In mid-August, to celebrate Cathy's thirty-ninth Birthday, we took several couples to dinner at a Thai restaurant in Noyack, NY, which is about twenty minutes from our summer home. It was there that Cathy surprised us all—in addition to wearing a tight little black dress that showed off her newly sculpted body, tan legs and arms, she wore no wig and no bandana. Her short, short hair seemed very chic, like Halle Berry. Her breasts were large and firm because the insides were still filled with oversized tissue expanders. She felt and looked like a beautiful woman for the first time in nine months.

As she walked into the restaurant, men looked at her the way men look at a beautiful young woman. I couldn't believe that just six months earlier she was gaunt, bald, felt mutilated and was virtually too sick to even talk. Once again, I had a fireball of energy in my house who was the epitome of kindness and thoughtfulness—proof positive that the human body is resilient and the human spirit is indefatigable. When Cathy underwent her mastectomies, I had emailed our friends that she was tough as nails and would rise to any challenge, and I was right. She didn't conquer chemo, but she faced it, endured it, let it work its necessary evils on her system and came away healthier, albeit with some long-term but manageable damage to her system. The alternative was to run a greater risk of recurrence and possible metastasis, which would have been unthinkable.

Cathy and I understand that chemotherapy is a necessary part of the curing process. You suffer through it one day at a time—hopefully, with a powerful support system at your side. We called our chemotherapy support system our "chemo team," which was made up of Cathy's friends—Kim (especially Kim), Jill, Janie, Caryl, Janet, Christine, Nancy, Leslie, Donna, Debbie, Marty, Andrea, Katie, Amy, Iona, Linda, Melinda and Judy. These wonderful women made Cathy's life, my life and our kids' lives much easier during a difficult time. Whether it was holding Cathy's hand during a chemo session or picking up Brandon for a play date and dinner, they were there for us. I learned that my wife was a quality friend by seeing and feeling the sincere outpouring of love and concern from her friends.

Our parents were also there for us, whenever we needed them. While my mother-in-law suffered vicariously with her daughter, she constantly supported her with a form of strength that can only come from Mommy. Our parents came for visits or didn't come—they complied with our requests, so we never had too much company, or company at the wrong time. Their visits and phone calls were effective because they surrounded Cathy, me and, more importantly, Brandon and Ryan with the type of support that showed us that we were not in this alone, despite the considerable physical distance between us.

Although the chemo was brutal on Cathy, we knew that we were lucky because she didn't need radiation treatments as well. We were acutely aware of how much more abuse women take when they have to endure chemo and radiation. For as bad as things got, they could have been worse, because radiation simply prolongs the abuse heaped on a woman when she is battling breast cancer.

CHAPTER 6
RECONSTRUCTIVE SURGERY

After Cathy's bilateral mastectomies, we learned during follow-up visits with both the reconstructive plastic surgeon and the breast surgeon that Cathy would be physically recovered from the surgery in about four weeks. We would then schedule regular visits with Dr. Disa's office for periodic expansions of the tissue expanders. We also learned that the expanders would come out in September and be replaced with permanent implants. This operation is referred to as "the transfer." It could have been done sooner than September, but no surgery can be scheduled during chemotherapy because the patient would be too weak. Besides, Cathy would also need time to recover from chemo and restore her immune system—and we had made the important decision during post—surgery adjuvant chemotherapy that she would have a prophylactic oophorectomy, a surgery to remove a woman's ovaries. It seemed like an obvious choice; the toxicity of Cathy's chemotherapy agents had rendered her ovaries useless, and since she likely carried the BRAC-2 gene, she could have as high as a 15 percent chance of developing ovarian cancer during her lifetime. Since all that Cathy's ovaries could give her was ovarian cancer, there was no need for her to have them anymore. The logical sequence for this second surgery was concurrent with "the transfer," as it would limit the risks associated with surgery.

We arranged to have Richard Baracat, a gynecological surgeon who came highly recommended, perform this surgery and coordinate his schedule so that when he finished, Dr. Disa could work on Cathy's breasts. After scheduling this operation, we read a New York magazine article written about Dr. Baracat. Unbeknownst to us at the time, he was the head of gynecological surgery at MSKCC and regarded as the top gynecological surgeon in New York City—which, as typical New Yorkers, we interpreted to mean one of the best in the world! In addition to his impressive credentials, he is a caring and kind man with a robust but dry sense of humor.

The recovery from "the transfer" and the oophorectomy is about three weeks. However, it isn't a totally miserable three weeks—your mental outlook is much better than when recovering from the mastectomies with the prospect of beginning four months of chemotherapy. "The transfer" is cosmetically enhancing while the oophorectomy is meant to ensure that cancer won't come back. The notion that when you heal you will look and be better able to move on with the rest of your life is really important; by contrast, after the mastectomies in January, all we had to look forward to was a cold winter, chemotherapy, more surgery and uncertainty.

"The transfer," or replacement of tissue expanders to permanent implants, is an intricate and lengthy procedure which Cathy underwent on September 25, 2003. Dr. Disa opened the horizontal incision scars where the nipples had been, then cut the pectoralis muscle vertically, which accessed the fully expanded, saline filled tissue expanders. He drained the expanders and removed them from the "capsule" that Cathy's body had created within her chest cavity over the previous seven months. He then inserted another set of implants into the newly created capsule, which he filled with silicone. We chose silicone as opposed to saline because they are softer and more natural looking, and we were convinced—after significant research—that they were safe. Dr. Disa next shaped the breasts by internally suturing the excess skin from Cathy's previously over—expanded breasts. Because of this internal suturing, the new permanent breasts are slightly smaller than the fully expanded tissue expander—filled breasts. They are however, more symmetrical and significantly more natural looking, as the surgeon has the opportunity to create a natural sag and carefully defined cleavage. Once this operation is complete, all that is left are two modest procedures.

Dr. Disa also performed the next procedure on September 16, 2004, in which he created nipples and areolae. While this was cosmetic surgery, it still took two hours, but because it went exactly as planned, it seemed exceptional. While many women choose not to have this surgery done at all, we learned that the younger the patient, the higher the probability that they will elect to have nipple and areola construction.

The first step of this operation, which was done under general anesthetic, was to "pinch" and suture the skin on the parts of Cathy's breasts that were farthest away from her body, in order to create nipples. Once this was done, Dr. Disa took a small amount of skin from Cathy's tummy and used it as a graft to create areolas. Many surgeons use excess skin from the fold of a woman's groin because that skin is darker and more naturally matches the coloration of a woman's areola. We elected to use the skin from Cathy's tummy because we were advised that the recovery process would go much faster than using the skin from her groin. Our thinking was that since she would need to have her nipples tattooed a darker pigment at a later time; she may as well have the areolas tattooed then as well, which is both a common and recommended approach.

A week after the surgery, when I accompanied Cathy to Dr. Disa's office for the removal of the post-surgical dressing, I was really amazed by the results. Cathy's surgically created nipples and areolas looked completely like "real ones." This is not always the case. Reconstructive surgery is sometimes limited by the quantity and quality of skin and tissue that remains after breast surgery and treatment. Furthermore, the amount and elasticity of skin will vary from patient to patient. In many instances, the elasticity of a woman's skin is compromised by radiation treatments. Radiation, another important tool in the fight against cancer, is a localized treatment whereby a beam of radiation is fired into the area that still could contain cancer cells. The hope is to eliminate and prevent a local recurrence of the disease. Radiation is a local therapy and differs from chemotherapy, which is a systemic therapy. And although radiation is generally less debilitating than chemotherapy, the radiation beams can damage the skin like a burn, diminishing its elasticity and making it more challenging for the reconstructive surgeon to achieve superior cosmetic results.

While women's nipples ordinarily change posture or shape as a result of heat, cold, sexual stimulation, as well as during lactation, surgically reconstructed nipples will not. Cathy and I naturally wondered what posture the surgeon would create on the new nipples. Would he give us a choice? Actually, the nipples immediately after surgery and for the next six months are completely erect, as if the woman had just walked out of an icy-cold pool. Over time, starting at about six months, they start to "settle" into a natural position, which is about halfway between a warm bath and icy pool. Creating the permanent posture of the nipples takes about a year and is as much of an art as any other aspect of the surgery.

At the time of this writing, Cathy has not yet been back for her tattooing, though we expect that this will complete the look and provide both of us with physical and emotional comfort.

There are many different types of surgery for breast cancer, and as the spouse of a woman with the disease, I believe it is important to learn everything you can about whatever surgical options might be appropriate, and to be certain that whatever choice you make is consistent with your ultimate goal. Our goal was disease-free survival. While we were very aggressive in the pursuit of our goal, I realize that our goal may not be correct for everyone, based on your overall health and age. You should try to chose a surgery team and hospital that both understands and is capable of handling your needs, with the thought that your needs may change considerably. Too many patients say, "I'll go to my local community hospital because my problem isn't so serious yet. If things get bad, I can always to go to a cancer center or large teaching hospital." Cathy and I feel strongly that nobody with cancer should wait for things to "get serious" before seeking out experienced and competent cancer specialists.

We frequently repeat that cancer surgery is not a commodity service, as there are immense qualitative differences not only in surgeons, but also in surgery techniques, nursing, pathology labs, and oncology. Ideally, denial and money should not get in the way of having the surgery performed correctly the first time, because cancer can be a very aggressive disease and should be treated as such. When we learned that Cathy needed a mastectomy, it was devastating, but in hindsight, it isn't nearly as bad or life altering, as we initially feared. If you have a question about a procedure, ask it, and don't move on until you get an answer you understand. You cannot be expected to make good decisions and be completely supportive if your doctors are compartmentalizing information.

Finally, many times the outcome of surgery dictates the need for chemotherapy. However, many times it does not. Your ordeal may be close to over when your wife has surgery… and she may ultimately end up with very aesthetically appealing breasts and a more resilient, fresher outlook on life. It is key for a loving and supportive husband to stay focused and organized so that you and your wife can set realistic goals and systematically achieve them.

CHAPTER 7

SEX AND INTIMACY

Intimacy before, during and after breast cancer is a topic that women talk about with each other and in support groups. Men however, generally feel uncomfortable discussing these issues, and often don't have outlets to express their feelings. I believe that men feel guilty for wondering about the sexual consequences of cancer when they think they should be totally focused on their wife's survival and mental well being. It's because of this guilt that most men just suffer in silence, refusing to bring up their concerns or insecurities about their needs and desire for sex and intimacy.

My sex life with Cathy has always been very good and never really taken much "work"; we always had a natural attraction that morphed into a loving, natural affection. Furthermore, our channels of communication were always good when it came to sex and intimacy. One of my early thoughts when I found out that Cathy had cancer was a fear that an important part of our marriage would be harmed or even lost. For many years, I've heard people make negative comments about their sex lives with their wives. Often, these comments were cloaked in jokes or funny stories, but I felt pity for a lot of these men because they characterized their intimacy with their wives with comments like "I got some" as if the enjoyment of intimacy was only one-sided.

I was fortunate on several fronts, as it was Cathy who would often initiate lovemaking, which was almost always mutually satisfying. Was this going to change? Was I going to feel like one of the complainers from my peer group? Was such a beautiful part of our life together going to collapse or disappear? Would I look for intimacy elsewhere? Would I find myself just going through the motions of sex in a perfunctory manner? Would Cathy? These questions really bothered me because I wasn't sure about the answers. And I felt that if I were to verbalize these concerns to anyone while Cathy's survival was still in question, I would be considered callous with priorities that were simply wrong. Therefore, I was on my own to figure out much of this over the course of the weeks and months after Cathy's diagnosis.

I also had no idea what the results of Cathy's mastectomies, chemotherapy and oophorectomy would have on her emotional and physical desires for intimacy. Nobody had told me what to expect—not because they didn't know, but rather because the concern with treating a cancer patient is to cure them. The sexual needs of their spouse generally—and understandably—get overlooked.

Further complicating my thinking was that Cathy's breasts may not have been central to, but had always played a part in our sex life. I found myself uncomfortably wondering that without the pleasure sensors in her breasts, would I be able to satisfy my wife? After all, reconstructed breasts are aesthetically appealing, but not subject to the sort of stimulation of a woman's natural breasts. I've never heard another man talk about giving sexual pleasure to his own wife because it is considered "crossing the line" with regard to respect and openness. In addition, most women who are diagnosed with breast cancer are already post-menopausal so they and their partner have already experienced the related impact of menopause and the diminution of sexual desire that often accompanies it. And the menopausal process happened over a period of time. Cathy, at thirty-eight-years old, had not experienced menopause, nor had most of her friends. During chemotherapy, her ovaries basically stopped functioning because of the toxicity of the drugs, which were a prelude to September 2003, when she underwent the prophylactic oophorectomy.

This operation, designed to prevent ovarian cancer and a possible recurrence of breast cancer, resulted in menopause becoming a sudden event rather than a gradual process.

The sexual component of our life came into focus very early during our cancer experience. I remember holding Cathy in bed the night before her initial surgery, while neither of us could sleep because we were petrified about the pain and uncertainty that the next day would bring. When I told her I wanted to make love to her, she pulled away. Rather than accept that and just turn over and go to sleep, I opened my heart and expressed all of my fears (except the part of looking for intimacy elsewhere) and concerns about our love life. I told her how much I treasured our intimacy and that I wanted to always treasure it. We both acknowledged that it would take a tremendous amount of work for her to be comfortable with herself and for me to be comfortable with her.

I felt confident that as I showed complete acceptance of Cathy after surgery, as well as during and after chemo, she would begin to feel more secure about herself. My goal was to make her feel sexy and desirable, even in the face of having surgically altered, not—yet reconstructed breasts, and being gaunt and bald. We made love that night, and for the first time ever during sex, I did not touch her breasts. I couldn't bring myself to do it, knowing that they wouldn't be there the next morning. Nevertheless, it was a tender, open and satisfying experience as we were more intimate than sexual. Without speaking it, we acknowledged to each other how important this aspect of our lives had always been. At that point, we were guessing that our love life would be challenged only by surgery and possibly by chemotherapy. Neither of us understood the consequences of a sudden menopause combined with estrogen suppressing medications like Arimidex, or estrogen blocking agents like Tamoxifen, both of which are part of the post treatment!

When Your Wife Has Breast Cancer

I was very fortunate that we had a strong marriage with very deep roots before cancer, and was doubly fortunate in that my love and respect for my wife grew considerably during the entire ordeal. Cathy faced her cancer as bravely and openly as she could; she used a degree of denial to protect herself, but in general was completely accepting of her new reality. Without ever admitting it, I know she was facing her illness more stoically than I could have if I were diagnosed with cancer. Her constant concern wasn't for herself, but rather for her children and me. I saw the way she valiantly and selflessly moved into and through the world of cancer, and I was inspired by her strength.

This inspiration fueled an attraction to Cathy as a person that transcended any weirdness that I might have felt while my wife was temporarily robbed of her femininity. As I perceive it, a woman's femininity is defined by three external aspects: her hair, breasts and hips. While this malicious disease was going to temporarily rob Cathy of two of those elements, it was also taking them from my wife, which meant that I too, though on a much lesser level, was being robbed.

On Dr. Heerdt's rather emphatic advice, we made love a few weeks after surgery, right before she started chemotherapy. It was hard for us both, physically and emotionally. Physically, because we were both tense and nervous, and emotionally, because we still had no idea what the future would hold in this area.

During chemotherapy, however, sex understandably was not on the forefront of Cathy's mind, since she felt like hell for about nine out of the fourteen days between cycles. On the first good day of the third two-week cycle, we actually had a really nice day together. It was one of those days when we both saw the world in really positive terms, which was hard to do because external events were really starting to press on us. It was an unusually cold winter, our country was about to go to war, our economy was in a sorry state, my oldest son was depressed because his surgically repaired knee was healing slowly, and most importantly, our boys Brandon and Ryan were suffering through Cathy's cancer.

When Cathy came to bed that night, she did something that I will never forget. She took off her bandana and then her shirt, confidently and bravely. She was willing to "present" herself to me so openly and fully at a time when she had large scars on both breasts, and the breasts themselves were very small because she was still at the beginning of the expansion process. She no longer had the extra confidence that her long blonde hair and petite lovely body had always given her. Her comfort with me and with herself made it exceptionally easy for me to be both loving and accepting.

The sex that night was really beautiful and intimate, and I felt as though my love for Cathy had reached new heights. My overpowering feelings of love and respect made the sex extremely intense and satisfying, which was remarkable because it was probably at the lowest point of Cathy's physical appearance. I remember thinking how lucky I was to be in love with my wife, and knew that I could and would be attracted to her no matter how she physically appeared. And I wanted to make her feel desirable and sexy, because to me, she was both. I was pleasantly surprised that I was able to disregard the vicious external changes to her body and see only a beautiful woman. Yet, despite my total acceptance of Cathy's appearance, I remained optimistic and certain that she would emerge from this entire ordeal without too much physical scarring. I focused on the fact that one day I would be able to look at my wife and not be reminded of the disease that had ravaged her body.

Everyone describes breast reconstruction after mastectomies as restorative surgery for a woman. I agree that it is, but it is also restorative to her husband because it restores a physical element of femininity that was viciously taken away. Cathy's reconstruction centered around the "expansions" she went through at the reconstructive surgeon's office. Generally, our plastic surgeon didn't do these expansions; they were done by one of his two very competent nurses. During these visits, Cathy would lie on the examination table and one of the nurses would use a magnet to find the metal ring that surrounded the rubber aperture of the implant, which was creating a new cavity inside Cathy's chest. Once found, the nurse would draw a circle around it on Cathy's skin with a marker, then insert a needle into the circle that would penetrate through the skin, the muscle under the skin and through the rubber aperture. The needle would then be attached to a syringe, which would be used to inject saline into the expanders.

Simply put, Cathy's breasts grew larger during each expansion. The first time I watched them get expanded, it reminded me of Bruce Banner becoming the Hulk! It wasn't long until they were larger than they had been before cancer. The tissue expanders aren't the most perfectly shaped implants, but they looked like large, firm breasts when covered in clothing. This gave Cathy a degree of confidence and kept my healthy state of denial intact.

My denial was pretty straightforward; I wanted my wife to ultimately look every bit as sexy, and perhaps, even sexier than she was before cancer. This was typical of how I approached life; I had exerted a sense of denial into a process that was larger than me and well beyond my control. I defiantly latched onto to this hope/expectation, even though I knew that I would love and accept my wife no matter what this disease did to her appearance.

As Cathy managed chemo and the expansions took hold, my sense of denial regarding the long-term physical impact of cancer became validated because her external beauty and vibrancy returned. While her hair grew back and she grew healthier and more beautiful, I kept noting how she was getting closer to the magical point of pre-cancer. This desire to return to conditions before her cancer diagnosis was just another form of denial. I rationalized it as my "stubborn optimism," but it was a way of protecting my fragile psyche from the present by coating it with a vision of the future that I found not only acceptable, but also appealing. It helped me block out the facts that Cathy was struggling for survival—her chest had endured a traumatic, invasive and temporarily disfiguring surgery, and she was being bombarded with chemotherapy that was wreaking havoc on her system. I needed to believe that I would wake up one day and it would all be over, that Cathy would be "as good as new." I didn't share my own little mind games with anyone because they would wonder how I could focus on my own "shallow" sexual or vanity needs at such an inappropriate time.

Upon reflection, my shallow needs were fueled in part by my own sense of narcissism, as I was acutely aware of how pleasing it was for me to be seen with a beautiful wife. I had always taken pleasure in the admiring looks Cathy received from men in our social circle, and I didn't want that to change. And I certainly didn't want to be on the receiving end of anyone's pity. On more than one occasion I thought, *When Cathy is outwardly beautiful again they can shove their pitiful looks and thoughts up their asses.* Cathy's appearance always addressed her sense of vanity, but also validated mine. I considered my feelings on this topic and guessed that they were common to many men in my position, but weren't expressed because most men don't want to seem shallow and self-absorbed. Perhaps I was so attuned to these feelings and because I was pretty secure within myself… or perhaps I was—and am—extremely shallow and self-absorbed? I guess it depends on whom you ask.

I was scheduled to attend a support group for husbands at Memorial Sloan Kettering Cancer Center, and looked forward to hearing about those feelings from other men who were supporting wives going through the same treatments as Cathy. I assumed that in the confines of a support group, these sorts of feelings would come out with a sense of understanding that only men in comparable positions could feel. I had never been to any kind of support group, but thought that a support group would be a safe place for frank and open dialogue.

The support group for husbands was facilitated by Roz Kleban, a very capable social worker who also facilitated MSKCC's support groups for women. I was certain that this group would discuss their feelings of cancer's impact on intimacy and expected to learn about their experiences to the extent that their wives went through sudden and premature menopause. I simply didn't think that the support group's only focus would be on acute issues like chemotherapy protocols and survival statistics. I wanted and expected the group to cover the day-to-day issues, the sub-acute issues, that husbands of breast cancer patients were experiencing. I guess my expectations were somewhat unrealistic, because I got hammered at my first and only support group meeting!

There were about ten of us at the table when Roz asked each of us to bring up something that we felt was important and wanted to share. The guys ranged in age from forty to about sixty-five. To Roz's great credit, she arranged the group so that all men had wives with either stage IIA or IIB breast cancer, which meant that they were living with or had lived with chemotherapy that included the drug Cathy referred to as "the red devil," Adriamycin.

The guys for the most part talked candidly and emotionally about their experiences with chemo or with surgery. One guy spoke about his wife's cancer being misdiagnosed at another hospital and his feelings of frustration and guilt for not questioning the doctor who initially screwed up. To my discredit, I didn't read the room correctly; this group was focused on the survival of their spouses, the acute issues, and I should have respected this. No one in the group really spoke about the private things that I felt only husbands in our situation could really feel. Sexuality had to be one of those items, yet the discussions didn't go there.

When it was my turn, I took a chance and spoke about my desire to know what type of breasts my wife would end up having after the reconstruction process, thinking that this would start a discussion about the sexual consequences of cancer treatments. The guy to my right began radiating hostility at me for initiating this type of discussion. He was about sixty years old and probably thinking that I was a shallow, uncaring little SOB whose paramount and only concern should have been my wife's survival.

This guy actually interrupted me twice, stating that his love for his wife far outweighed something as petty as the appearance of her breasts. He seemed to hold sway with the room because I felt it was eleven (including Roz) against one. I suddenly identified with Henry Fonda in *Twelve Angry Men*! His hostility also sparked my sense of defiance, as I defended myself by telling the group that I loved my wife completely, and was focused both on her recovery and survival and on protecting my kids. I also pointed out that every time I went to the reconstructive plastic surgeon's office and looked at his book of pictures of reconstructed breasts, I saw pictures of overweight, post-menopausal women with youthful looking breasts that didn't quite fit. I wanted to see pictures of young, beautiful women with reconstructed breasts because my wife is young and beautiful. I explained that if the new breasts weren't going to be beautiful, then I wanted to start coming to grips with that now and not be disappointed later.

My comments, which must have made me sound like a spoiled child, opened up a flood of scorn, derision and hostility from the group—especially from the guy to my right. He even scolded me, saying that he loved his wife unconditionally and that I would be well advised to reorient my priorities. At this point, having taken enough of his shit, I looked him squarely in the eyes and said that my love for my wife has gotten us through thirteen years of marriage, that it wasn't for him to judge on a qualitative basis, and that wanting to know what sort of breasts would press against my body for the rest of our lives was a fair concern because it was one of my concerns. I then weakly added that reconstruction wasn't only for the woman's benefit!

Fortunately, another guy in the group, Richard, came to my defense and said that he understood why I was not prepared to let go of the image of a stunning and beautiful wife. Richard lived near us and had actually met Cathy and me during happier times. His wife is also young and beautiful, and went through surgery and chemo over the last year. I'm grateful that he took me out of the hot seat that night.

After the meeting, Richard and I walked uptown together and had a pretty open conversation about sex and intimacy, and it actually validated my feelings of concern. It also validated my feelings that it was OK to hope to have an even more beautiful and happy wife at the end of treatments and surgery. During the fifteen block walk, Richard took me from feeling like an uncaring piece of garbage to feeling like a normal man with normal concerns. I felt very lucky to have the opportunity to speak so candidly with someone, and I was very happy that he was able to lift my spirit after such an uncomfortable experience.

For the next few months, I tried to evaluate all the thoughts that were going through my head regarding our future life together, and part of that thinking centered on intimacy. Fortunately, as we progressed through chemo and saw that Cathy was responding to it in a manner that pleased her oncologist, I began to think of the rest of our lives together as a long time. After she finished Adriamycin (the first eight weeks of chemo), she moved onto a drug called Taxol. Since she was significantly less miserable on Taxol than Adriamycin, we could focus a little more on intimacy. Additionally, Cathy's pain from her surgery had lessened, which made sex less physically demanding. Unfortunately, she was still bald, which was troublesome to both of us. Many women come to accept baldness during chemotherapy and become less bothered by it as time passes. Cathy never got to that point, and we both started to really hate the wigs, turbans and bandanas. I put all my effort into making her feel desirable by asking her not to wear any head covering in bed and kissed her head frequently. I don't know what affect this had on Cathy, but I suspect it was positive.

I have heard several instances of men either not seeing their wives' bodies after surgery or not seeing their wives' heads while they were bald. I understand this on some level, but strongly discourage it. I saw Cathy's breasts before she was ready to show them to me when I attempted to adjust her position in bed, just three days after her surgery. It was startling for me, but in retrospect, I'm glad I saw them when I did; I knew that they wouldn't get any worse, and at the time Cathy was too physically uncomfortable to be self-conscious. When I saw Cathy's breasts after "the transfer," which exchanged the tissue expanders for permanent implants, they were absolutely beautiful. They were natural looking, symmetrical and looked as if they belonged on Cathy. My initial optimism about the postsurgical cosmetic outcome had been surprisingly correct, and a year later, when Dr. Disa completed the nipple and areola construction, Cathy's breasts became more beautiful still.

I'm not sure how Cathy braced herself for the possibility that her reconstruction might not turn out well, but I prepared myself by grasping for information about the process. I didn't want to show disappointment upon seeing Cathy's breasts because I knew that my approval would be key to her acceptance of her own appearance. As it turned out, neither of us was disappointed.

From a sexual point-of-view, I thought the aftermath of Cathy's surgery and chemotherapy would be the only really difficult parts. Unfortunately, I totally underestimated the sexual and psychological effects of premature menopause. Chemotherapy treatments are designed to kill the cancer cells, but they also suppress the production of estrogen as breast cancer cells feed on estrogen. Estrogen is created in the ovaries, which typically shut down (many times permanently) from the chemo. This shutting down of ovarian function, known as menopause, has its own very pronounced impact on female sexuality, all of it negative. Cathy's ovaries shut down during chemotherapy, but that was largely irrelevant since her ovaries were removed four months after chemo had ended. At thirty-eight-years old, Cathy was in menopause and wasn't ready for it. Neither was I.

We are only now learning how to cope with this from a sexual viewpoint. When chemo shut down Cathy's ovaries (this doesn't always happen and can be avoided if a patient wants to have children later), she was thrust into a world of hot flashes, diminished sex drive, night sweats, and unfortunately, vaginal dryness. The diminution of estrogen causes a thinning of the vaginal lining and inhibits the vagina's ability to lubricate itself while aroused. This vaginal dryness, combined with a lack of interest in sex, was and remains challenging. We are learning to work through all of this, which isn't easy, but compared to the rigors of cancer, isn't tragic.

When I was a child, my father often used a phrase that I never fully grasped when speaking about problems. He would say, "Mark, when you are up to your ass in alligators, you don't complain about getting your pants wet." This sums up sex and cancer. When it is unclear if your spouse will survive, you cannot focus too much attention on sex. The only unfortunate part of this is that after your wife is "out of the woods" on the survival front, sex somehow gets lost in the transition, which is a shame—men want sex before cancer and will still want it afterward, and they shouldn't be made to feel guilty for that.

Cathy's hot flashes and night sweats are actually going away quickly because of the tremendous amount of exercise that she does daily. I don't know when or if the diminished sex drive will be completely overcome, but seeing as I have no choice and treasure our marriage, I'll wait and be optimistic because optimism is in my DNA. The vaginal dryness is tricky business—it isn't just the dryness of initial penetration, as that can be overcome with some simple topical lubricant like KY jelly. Rather, it is a significant drop in mucous and other natural vaginal lubrication, which causes irritation and pain during sex. The application of a topical lubricant only accommodates easier initial penetration.

In order to compensate for this problem, Cathy's oncologist inserted into her vagina, an estring, a device which releases a small localized dose of estrogen, which in turn lubricates itself. The estring, much like an IUD, cannot be felt during intercourse, and since it releases only a small amount of estrogen that's contained in the vagina, it doesn't increase a woman's risk of further cancer.

It is ironic that we find ourselves happy, in love, confident and attracted to each other physically, yet we are having a moderate degree of trouble with sex. This isn't too upsetting because we are confident that we can work through it. I am also certain that other post-menopausal women have figured out how to work around the discomfort of their symptoms and can enjoy sex and intimacy with their partners. We are confident of being able to get through this because we got through the much more difficult stages of having intimacy and sexual relations immediately after surgery and during chemo. We both accepted Cathy's appearance at those difficult times as a temporary setback because of our love for each other and our optimistic view of the future. I made love to my wife when she was gaunt, surgically impaired and bald, so dealing with some vaginal dryness and other menopausal discomforts is easy by comparison.

I've spoken with other men whose wives have had breast cancer and have had similar experiences to mine. Their feelings about sex have been surprisingly upbeat, with only a few of them saying that their sex lives have suffered over the long term. Each of them did explain, however, that they experienced varying degrees of difficulty during the short term. Generally, while the men were hesitant to admit it at first, they felt that the reconstructed breasts were at least as appealing aesthetically as their wives' original breasts. Most of the men who felt this way have been ill at ease discussing this with their spouses, but all noted that their wives enjoy the appearance of their "new," firm breasts.

One man said that he had particular trouble making love or being intimate with his wife while she was bald and undergoing reconstruction. In fact, he had trouble looking at her naked. I asked him if he felt this was his doing or his wife's, and he answered that he took his cues from his wife, as she was never comfortable with herself and her discomfort made him both awkward and uncomfortable. It was only after about a year after her chemo was over, her hair was largely back (she always had short hair) and her reconstruction was mostly complete that she let him back into her life physically, emotionally and sexually. He struck me as a laid-back type who wasn't terribly upset by the hiatus in their intimacy. He said he was pretty confident the whole time that it would eventually come back. I admired this attitude and learned that sexual problems that have arisen from cancer are solvable, but take time as well as understanding to resolve.

While cancer can rob a person of their external looks, it cannot rob someone of their internal beauty, and it is in this internal beauty that I discovered my true love for Cathy. This love has lead to some very satisfying lovemaking because my attraction to my wife was deeper and more powerful than ever before. This has left me hopeful that as she moves farther away from surgery and chemotherapy, both her internal and external beauty will drive our lovemaking. Not only am I hopeful about this, but I'm positive about it. Perhaps this is another example of my denial sustaining my sense of optimism, but I also believe that Cathy's love for and trust in me will have grown, and her feelings about me will blossom, which will ultimately fuel her passion and sexual enjoyment.

CHAPTER 8

THE PERSONAL FINANCES OF BREAST CANCER

"Money, money… is that all you ever think about?" I must have been asked this question a hundred times in my adult life, which is really ridiculous—if a man doesn't focus on or make much money, or he's an irresponsible spender, then he isn't considered a good provider. And while society has somehow inculcated us with the notion that good providers are generally good husbands, if you talk about money as it relates to your wife's cancer right after she is diagnosed, you stand a good chance of being branded a bad husband or worse, a greedy SOB.

This is somewhat absurd because money can actually help you and your wife get through breast cancer with a better chance of surviving it intact! While having money won't save your wife's life from a cancer that's absolutely determined to kill her, it may help you save her life if the cancer is remotely curable. Furthermore, having money will afford you more choices in healthcare, plus allow you to be there physically as well as emotionally to support your wife and children during the battle, because there are times when she will be challenged and may want to stop fighting.

Unfortunately, there is a pretty strong chance that your wife's breast cancer will wreak havoc on your personal finances, regardless of whether or not you have money. If you have little or no savings, this disease just adds insult to injury. If you have a decent financial cushion, this disease will wreck it. Only the really rich will not become financially battered, and since most families aren't super rich—including the Weiss family—most will suffer financially as well as emotionally and physically.

There are three primary ways that your wife's cancer can affect you financially:

1. Lost earnings at work.
2. The ancillary costs of the disease that you generally will have to pay for on an after tax basis.
3. Unreimbursed medical expenses.

For me, the enormity of lost wages was by far the most serious aspect of financial pain. However, the other two components, ancillary costs and uncovered medical bills, were also surprisingly severe. As I had no idea what these costs would be (though my gut instinct told me they were going to be significant), I took financial action three days after Cathy's diagnosis. I refinanced the mortgage on my apartment (I was lucky rates had dropped) and simultaneously expanded my home equity credit line against my second home. Because I am financially conservative, I needed to justify to myself that it was OK to borrow money to cover emergencies... and having a wife diagnosed with a potentially fatal and certainly debilitating disease, definitely qualified as an emergency!

Unfortunately, the time to start preparing financially for an emergency like cancer in your family is years before anyone gets sick. Too many people wait until bills overwhelm them before they realize that not only are they in a medical crisis, but in a financial one as well. I've been advising my close friends lately that they should prepare a financial emergency plan while everything in their life is good. This is such simple advice and so perfectly obvious to me now; however, unlike drafting a will or buying life insurance, most people have no financial emergency plan. I didn't. Whatever plan a person drafts without pressure will be better than one that is drafted under emotional duress and time consideration.

The Personal Finances Of Breast Cancer

Lost Earnings and a Damaged Career

Many men—assuming they are the providers in their family—feel tremendously guilty for focusing on money as soon as the day their wives are diagnosed with cancer. I was one of these men. I thought that my concern about affording the consequences of Cathy's cancer would negatively impact my ability to focus on the human consequences. When Cathy's cancer diagnosis came, I was six months into a new job and had tremendous positive momentum from stimulating work in a new environment that brought thirteen-hour days... no two being identical. Right up until her diagnosis, I was working productively with intensity and complete client focus. Suddenly, I was confronted with a colossal "distraction," which I knew right away would be bad for business—both servicing existing business as well as developing new business.

Many men, and probably myself included, draw a fair amount of personal esteem from their professional success, and being financially productive is regarded as a metric of that esteem sustaining success. This isn't true in all fields, but it certainly is in mine—commercial real estate brokerage. I don't work just for money, but unfortunately, it is one of the things that others use to judge my professional accomplishments. I've done intricate and innovative deals, helped the American Red Cross find office space to support their crisis center after 9-11 (without taking a fee, of course,) and have lectured on ethics for the Real Estate Board of New York. Regardless, I am known more within my industry for financial success than for anything else I've been able to achieve over a twenty-one-year career.

For me, the prospect of not being able to work without distraction, which would cause me to make considerably less money, meant that I would lose standing within my industry. This is really pathetic, but true. Other jobs have their own separate currencies or indicators of success—a baseball player's may be hitting homeruns, while a surgeon's, is saving lives—

and while money is certainly a factor in measuring their success, I'm in a field where money transcends itself. It is how people measure themselves against their peers. I didn't fully realize this until Cathy got sick and my ability to earn was compromised.

My point is that if your wife or partner has breast cancer, many areas in your life will suffer, including your professional life, where you generate the currency that makes you successful. Having this currency, whatever it is, eroded by your wife's cancer is really upsetting as most men are too embarrassed to say that they resent cancer's intrusion into their professional success. First and foremost, every man whose wife is afflicted with breast cancer wants her to be healed and safe. However, society doesn't permit men to say things like, "I'm really pissed off that I missed out on a critical professional opportunity because I was sleep deprived and unfocused from being so overwhelmed with taking care of my kids and my sick wife." You can feel it, but you can't say it.

People who haven't lived through a spouse's cancer may think that the only major financial loss is un-reimbursed medical expenses. For me, the greatest single cost has been lost productivity at work. People who own their own business or work on a commission-only basis—better known as an "eat what you kill" environment—are really in trouble if they don't have an infrastructure to cover for them during the endless hours of downtime throughout the various stages of a spouse's illness. Remember, even if you are smart enough to have disability insurance, it doesn't cover you for not making a living because you're going from hospital to shrink, to plastic surgeon's office, to genetic counselor, to support group, to wig shop, to your kids' school (remember, during chemo your wife will be immunosuppressed, so she can't go to the school), to the pain management specialist, to the gastroenterologist, and to the oncologist's office.

For most people, being successful at work is the result of smarts and hard work. Consistent success, however, also requires inertia and rhythm. I always have different clients at various stages of the "deal cycle," meaning that I've nursed and developed some transactions for as long as four years and others for as short as six months. Invariably, I have some projects that are finishing, some starting, and others at points in between. This even pipeline of business leads to consistency in performance, and has provided me with the confidence and inertia that makes bringing in new business relatively easy. I never had to press to make a deal that didn't quite fit; I've always had a backlog of potentially profitable projects that I had generated, as I've always been able to focus on marketing myself and my firm. Each success increased my appetite for hard work and landing my next client. But Cathy's illness completely broke my inertia and rhythm, which beat my confidence to a pulp and distracted me to the extent that I could only concentrate intermittently on my work.

My thoughts became increasingly negative as my very certain little world quickly filled with uncertainty. People can sense when you are preoccupied or depressed; it comes out in very subtle ways, no matter how hard you try to mask it. This subtle negative energy can easily be the difference between getting hired by a prospective client or coming in second—and during the dark days of Cathy's illness, I came in second plenty! And unfortunately, there is no currency for coming in second.

Throughout the diagnostic and initial treatment phase of Cathy's illness, there were countless doctor's appointments, which I attended because Cathy and I faced the challenge of learning about the disease together. For my own medical care, I always hated it when a doctor double-booked and I had to spend more than fifteen minutes in their waiting room. I'd grumble, "Don't they teach doctors how to keep a schedule in medical school?" or "Maybe I should send him a bill for my time." Most people share their frustration with the nurses and secretaries in a medical office, but let the doctor off easily. Not me. I always let the doctor know that I held him or her accountable for keeping me waiting, which caused of them great discomfort when confronted about their lack of punctuality, or their callous disregard for their patients' time.

With my wife's illness, I couldn't be angry at any of her doctors. I knew that if we were kept waiting, they were likely with another patient, having a life-or-death discussion that may have been precipitated by a medical test they had just received. Consequently, we waited plenty and almost never got annoyed or complained. Only now, months later, do I shudder at the financial cost of my lost productivity while waiting with Cathy for those appointments. Then I would try to absorb everything the doctor said and not allow the appointment to move forward until I understood every detail (a practice which perhaps kept the next patient waiting). After a while, I stopped trying to calculate how much each frustrating doctor's appointment cost me. A thirty-minute appointment at 9:00 A.M. when we also had to wait thirty minutes to see the doctor generally took me out of a business mentality for half a day. I would leave the doctor's office, go to my office and try to squeeze a full day's worth of productivity into the other half of the day. Because I already "lost" half a day, I would unnaturally press for results, which was a recipe for consistent failure. I suddenly found myself in a position where I was working less, pressing harder, radiating a negative energy, and angry that I wasn't succeeding. Fortunately, it didn't take me long to realize that I needed to overhaul the way I was doing things and adjust my perspective on business success.

Each year, around November or December, I draft a personal business plan—a road map for how I am going to grow professionally, do better and more innovative work, take on better, higher—quality clients and assignments, and how I will contribute to my company and community. In mid-January 2003, I knew that I needed to revisit my recently completed business plan, and modify it by creating a six-month "life raft," which would be reserved for those deals and clients that were most important and had the highest probability of providing imminent financial reward. Because my capacity for work was diminished and would diminish further, I had to close my active deals, service my most important accounts, and be extra selective in pursuing new business.

On a professional level, my existing clients were as supportive and caring as I could have ever imagined. Fortunately (or miraculously), I didn't screw anything up for them during this crisis, and I learned that some of my long-term clients were really wonderful people. They reached out to my wife, my kids and me. Specifically, a few went way above and beyond my highest expectations during this time by comporting themselves more like friends than clients-among them, Corning Incorporated; Medical Liability Mutual Insurance Company, Inc.; Hartmarx Corporation; Country-Wide Insurance Company; Advent Software; Cornell University; Clarins USA; and SEIU 32BJ (New York City's largest union, and a relatively new client at the time).

Part of trying to focus my efforts more narrowly meant disengaging myself from some difficult situations. One particularly difficult client made extraordinary demands for my time and attention, which were disproportionate to the return available for completing a transaction with his company. He also had a very nasty edge whenever we spoke, which my assistant Halli, who has a very client-oriented, friendly demeanor, complained about several times. I remember calling "Russ" and telling him that his interests would be better served if he hired one of our competitors. He was stunned to be "fired" as a client, though not as stunned as I was to actually do it. I was relieved to have unburdened myself of this guy, but it reinforced the fact that I needed to accept that Cathy's illness was having a negative impact on my work life. Before she got sick, I would have handled this difficult client, or pretty much any other one, with relative ease. But now I just couldn't, and I was smart enough not to try because it would have been at the expense of other clients as well as my own sanity.

My new, streamlined business plan would be productive under my new circumstances, but would have a smaller yield than the model planned out in the business plan that I had just completed that past November. Simple translation: I would make less money in 2003 and needed to accept that quickly, or risk making no money in 2003!

One of my regrets for falling down professionally is that I am not the only one who relies on my productivity at work. Jeff Peck, a partner who is still learning the business and works closely with me on virtually all of my projects, tried as hard as he could to fill the void I created in our team, (and considering what he was up against, did a very credible job). While Jeff needed to get all of his own work done, he had to cover for me more and more, and step into some very intricate transactions without having had the benefit of structuring them from the beginning. I was proud of the way he stepped up to the added challenges, impressed with the results of his efforts and amazed that he never complained. Nevertheless, the financial consequence of my losing hours, days and weeks during the surgery and chemo had a negative financial impact on the Peck family as well as ours.

It is bizarre and awkward to admit, even to myself, but I was angry with Cathy. Her cancer had cost me the ability to provide for her and my boys, and disrupted my career, which was important to me—separate and apart from my family. I know this anger is terribly irrational, but in many ways, so are the lost earnings. Some people may compare them to an entire career of earnings, rather than just the previous year's. Half a year's worth of productivity against an entire career is modest; against 2003's total earnings, it is understandably steep. Therefore, I would argue that the financial impact varies greatly on perspective, and is psychologically easier if you adopt a long-term perspective, not unlike the one many investors take when their stocks suddenly lose value.

The Personal Finances Of Breast Cancer

For the most part, if you are candid with your colleagues and superiors at work, they will be supportive…to a point. Many of them, especially men, cannot understand, or even fathom the stress that you have at home. There is also a natural anger about your wife's cancer that can derail your career if you allow it to slip into your workplace. It can cause you to alienate the people you need to help pull you through this rough period. While I tried very hard to compartmentalize my home life and work life, I allowed my personal frustration to come out at work, more times than I care to admit.

I realize now that I was angry, thinking that my wife and partner in life might die prematurely, that she was suffering through treatments, which caused her to become bald and gaunt, and that my precious kids were suffering by watching her suffer. I believed my job at home was to absorb and ameliorate my family's frustrations, not to unburden myself by sharing mine with them. And my colleagues at work certainly weren't in a position to deal with my personal issues, particularly because I was relatively new and didn't have the longstanding, deep personal relationships that people form at work over time. The net result was that the people around me at work noticed that I had a black cloud over my head as they heard heated discussions (even behind closed doors) with lots of profanity coming out of my office.

Thinking back, if I wasn't so established in my industry, I could have been fired for much of my anger induced behavior, but since I had a track record of twenty years of "good behavior" and success, they assumed that the black cloud around me was only temporary. I wish I could have been calmer during this turbulent period because I knew that getting fired due to an anger induced breakdown would have lead to real financial pressure and crushed my self-esteem. I made Halli, my secretary, cry a couple of times, which still makes me wince because Halli wanted nothing more than to be helpful getting me through this. The truth is that she did a fantastic job.

Normally, if one of my colleagues missed a deadline on a project, it annoyed me and caused some frustration. But when Cathy was ill, if I had completed my portion of a project and the project stalled because someone else hadn't completed his or her task, I became outraged. I'd think, *I finished my end, and did it with diminished sleep, less time in the office and huge pressure at home. What's your excuse?* I recall snapping (maybe yelling) at Jeff Peck because he couldn't finish his end of a project in a timetable that I considered realistic. Not wanting to bother me, he hadn't kept me apprised of his progress, so I assumed nothing was wrong and that we were moving ahead. Therefore, I communicated an important delivery date to the client *without telling Jeff.* Compounding this problem was the fact that I was too preoccupied with cancer—related stuff to check on Jeff's progress. Additionally, when assigning tasks on the project, I wasn't clear enough about how something should be done and what the relative detail should include. Jeff, of course, assumed that his portion of the project needed tremendous detail. (It didn't).

I exploded, and in hindsight, realize that I was wrong on every front. Jeff may have made a mistake, but he had good intentions, and I gave him almost no direction. Just because Cathy had cancer and I was under strain didn't mean that people could read my mind, which I sort of expected Jeff to be able to do. I'm lucky that he was, and is, a compassionate person, and a good friend.

My office is next to my CEO's office, which is generally a good spot— except when you are ranting and raving about inconsequential things because you're walking around with a short fuse, feeling like your entire life is spinning out of control. One day in the middle of all this, my CEO, Barry Gosin, came into my office and closed the door. I fully expected to have my head handed to me for being too loud or too hard on people. It was right after I dropped my high-maintenance client and I was certain that it was coming back to haunt me. I assumed that Barry, who runs a company with 750 employees, was probably annoyed that he had to take time to give an attitude adjustment to one of his Executive Vice-Presidents. To my great surprise, he communicated his concern about Cathy and me, and reassured me that he knew I'd be able to pull through these difficult times. He urged me to recognize the warning signs before I lost my temper and to just come into his office and ask him to pinch-hit for me on any project, large or small. He ended his comments with "Mark, we are all here for you and will help you pull through this." I couldn't respond or even thank him, because if I uttered one syllable, I would have started to cry. I'll never forget his expression of support. I told Jeff about it and he restated the same thing. How lucky I was to be surrounded by these types of people.

The Ancillary Costs of Cancer

Very few people recognize the ancillary costs of cancer—these are the indirect costs related to the disease, as well as the disabling consequences of surgery and chemotherapy. If I were disabled for the better part of a year, I'd have the benefit of disability insurance, which is something very few women have and usually cannot get unless they are in the workforce. That was the case with us as we had life insurance on Cathy, but no disability insurance. Ideally, disability insurance would have compensated us for the cost of hiring people to do the things that Cathy did on a regular day. Many people think that I could have done some of the things that she typically did as a stay-at-home mom, but that wouldn't be putting my productive hours to their best financial use. Cathy's mother is in California, mine in Florida, my brothers live in London and Florida respectively, and Cathy's brother Jimmy is also in California. Family is the only reliable alternative to "Mom" unless you buy good, reliable help. So, we paid up and hired people to do much of Cathy's work at home. We were fortunate because the women we hired to help us through this difficult time were terrific.

Liz had been working for us only occasionally until Cathy got sick, but she was able to shift her class schedule at college to work for us five days a week. In addition to doing the cleaning and shopping, she helped Cathy during the darkest hours of her chemotherapy. She has the heart of a healer and made our lives easier. Liz was constant positive energy.

Maureen has worked for us as a babysitter for nine years. Her primary responsibility had been taking care of Ryan, but with Cathy's illness, her responsibilities increased dramatically. She took him to school each morning, picked him up in the afternoon and took him to play dates, doctor's appointments, haircuts… and all of the day-to-day things that a three-year old boy needs that Cathy typically would have done. Maureen was there for Cathy, me, Brandon and Ryan, and became an integral part of our household. She cemented herself as part of our family.

Unfortunately, we had a big void with Brandon. Cathy had typically focused an immense amount of time and energy on him, but suddenly was unable to do that. Our sensitive, now nine-year-old son needed someone to take him to doctor's appointments, play dates, Hebrew school, gymnastics and swimming plus help him with his homework. Cathy just couldn't do it and I couldn't truncate my already meager workday at 4:00 P.M., without further sacrificing my ability to financially support my family. This meant we needed to hire another person to work in our home from 3:00 P.M. to 8:00 P.M. each night. Liz's best friend Heather filled this role nicely. Her quiet demeanor and reliability were exactly what we needed. Our payroll for three basically fulltime people each week was staggering, but we really had no choice. We had to accept our new reality and be grateful that we could afford it.

On top of these ancillary costs, we had the added expense of psychiatric counseling. Insurance covers only a modest amount of therapy and we had plenty as Cathy, Brandon and I were in some sort of therapy, virtually every week. In fact, Cathy and I liked Brandon's shrink so much, we went to see him several times for joint counseling. The benefits of preserving our sanity and our ability to cope effectively were immense. These were in no way "luxuries"; rather, they were necessities that again, we were fortunate enough to be able to afford.

The mental health expense on top of the staggering weekly cost for additional household help caused my personal expense structure to climb at a time when making a living was severely challenged. Thankfully, I was able to anticipate this problem to a degree and put myself in a mental mindset whereby I looked at the initial six months of costs as extraordinary items. I was prepared to repay myself for these costs over 5 years and if need be, would have tapped my home equity line of credit to fund these 6 months. With this framework in place the financial enormity of our changed expense structure didn't bother me as much as I thought it would. I didn't like it, but appreciated that we were doing what we had to do and were in no way indulging in frivolous niceties to get past this period in our lives.

Wigs are another ancillary cost of cancer that surprised me, as the wig industry is nothing short of outrageous. A woman will generally need two wigs during chemotherapy; they need frequent service and adjustments and as one gets refitted and cleaned for a couple of weeks at a time, a woman can't walk around bald. Wigs are not cheap—they range in cost from $40 to $3,000. We got two at $1,000 each, which were a combination of synthetic and natural hair and looked good as far as wigs go. Fortunately, they came with a lot of service as Timothy, the stylist who sold them to Cathy, highlighted them and did all kinds of other crap (including talking to the wigs and calling them his "girls") to justify the high charge he presented to my wife as she was about to undergo chemotherapy.

When I first heard the price of wigs and learned that we needed two, I insisted that we go to Brooklyn on a Sunday morning to find some wig shop that catered to the Orthodox Jewish community to buy the second wig. I walked into a wig shop knowing exactly what we wanted because we already had one… and was treated like a lunatic with a can of spray paint in the Louvre. First, the women in the shop pretended they didn't speak English, then tried to get me to come back with an appointment for midweek—(without giving me their phone number). Finally, I looked the proprietor in the eye and said, "My wife has cancer, and you are humiliating me… I'll overpay for her wigs in Manhattan, but at least I'll get treated like a person." I think she was apologizing as I walked out of the store. I went back into the car where Cathy was waiting and said, "Let's go back to Manhattan, get ripped off and take it smiling." Our insurance company only reimburses for synthetic wigs, which look terrible.

Some costs go down during cancer—less dinners at restaurants, fewer hair colorings, less clothes shopping, vacations… hah! But some go up. Prepare for these costs as best as you can and try to mentally look at these extraordinary items in the context of your expense structure over a period of years. It will lessen the pain… a bit.

Unreimbursed Medical Costs

I touched on some indirect expenses and referred to them as ancillary costs. The direct costs that don't get covered by insurance are also pretty severe. Many people assume that medical insurance will protect your financial well-being during a medical catastrophe, but there are significant gaps in most insurances that will either have you fighting your insurance company or paying for a chunk of your wife's treatment with after-tax dollars. This assumes that you are fortunate enough to have insurance.

One of the first things I did was to speak to the head of Employee Benefits for my company and ask her to review with me what was covered and what wasn't. I wasn't thrilled with her responses, as they lacked specificity. It is amazing how a company benefits administrator will consider helping an employee deal with the blizzard of bills and confusing statements from hospitals and insurers to be "helping you with personal items."

My next call was to our insurer, who communicated what they would cover and what my deductibles and copays were, but made no mention about the gray area called "usual and customary." After our conversation, I was confident that my financial exposure would be capped at the maximum out-of-pocket per year/per insured of $10,000—the maximum deductible plus 20 percent of all physician and hospital costs because the hospital we chose was "out of network." The 20 percent is theoretically a capped number because we received more than $50,000 worth of medical treatment from MSKCC alone. Much of this was new to me; Cathy had always dealt with the medical stuff because most doctor's appointments were for our kids. Besides, I didn't worry because I assumed our maximum exposure as per the above was accurate based on conversations both with my insurance company and my benefits administrator at work.

As it turns out, I was dead wrong. In addition to the $10,000 of non-reimbursed medical costs, I was responsible for 100 percent of the amount of medical expenses that were denied by our insurer because they weren't "usual and customary," which to me is utter and complete nonsense. It allows an insurance company to determine what types of treatments are appropriate for an illness, and also permits them to dictate how much those treatments should cost. I live on the Upper East Side of Manhattan and chose a state-of-the-art cutting-edge cancer hospital to keep my wife alive. If I live in an area where it costs $495 a month to garage a car, how can an insurance company index medical costs in Manhattan to those in Binghamton, New York, where the costs are not nearly as severe? Furthermore, it costs more to attract doctors and nurses to Manhattan, as the cost of living is so high they need to be paid more. These costs must be passed through to the end user who needs to be backstopped by the insurance companies that should—and often times do—deal with the increased costs by adjusting the premium charges to the insureds. With the premiums adjusted to the location of the insureds, denying coverage citing "usual and customary" is a classic example of double-dipping by the insurance company to enhance their own profitability.

I can see where a policy needs to be set in place to safeguard against abuses by hospitals and doctors, but patients should have the right to seek the best possible medical care without having their insurance company telling them that they need to go to some cut-rate facility. We wanted the best physicians, using the latest medicine and technology, to cure an insidious disease. Since we chose to use an out-of-network hospital, I understood that I would be shouldering more of the burden of cost than if I used a hospital that had negotiated prices with our insurance company, and I was OK with this. In fact, I understand that our insurer wants to put up a deterrent for any of their insureds to utilize the more expensive healthcare providers by making the insured absorb up to 20 percent of the cost of this healthcare. However, selling a policy that features $10,000 per year of maximum exposure per insured, then looking for loopholes, is fundamentally unfair. I think that even my benefits coordinator at work was surprised when I explained to her that our policy uses a fuzzy concept like "usual and customary" to deter most insureds in major metropolitan areas from seeking and getting the best possible healthcare.

Since our insurer's definition of "usual and customary" differs greatly from MSKCC's definition, I found myself squarely in the middle of two large institutions locking horns over charges and reimbursements. I have been battling with the insurance company while maintaining a significant negative balance to MSKCC in the hopes of reducing my exposure to as close to $10,000 as possible. At the time of this writing, I am not terribly close to my goal, but still have a fair amount of fight in me. By withholding some monies to MSKCC while I duke it out with the insurer, I know that I can count on MSKCC's support in justifying why they did some of the things they did and why their charges for those services and procedures were, in fact, reasonable. I don't feel terrible about making MSKCC wait for payment because they have been paid for the vast majority of service provided, and because I learned that they, like most other hospitals, have a policy of charging higher rates to those with insurance in order to compensate for their significant losses in treating those without insurance. The Catch-22 is that insurance companies generally won't tolerate this sort of billing, which puts the insured in the position of covering the delta. In other words, people with insurance are asked to pay for those without insurance by paying higher premiums on their insurance and higher fees to hospitals. Although it is very difficult to consider all of the health implications in finding the right treatment for your wife while also figuring out how much that treatment will cost, you would be well advised to determine the answers to the following questions:

• What is the total likely cost and breakdown between surgeon's fee and hospital charges for your wife's surgery?

• What will the anesthesiologist charge for this operation?

• How much does your insurance company consider customary for the surgeon and anesthesiologist's fees as well as the hospital charges?

• What is the total likely cost of chemotherapy? Is chemo considered in-patient or out-patient, and what does your insurance company consider reasonable and customary for the purchase of drugs and their administration?

• What are the anticipated costs of reconstruction?

• Will silicone implants be covered, or only saline?

- Will your insurance company cap your reimbursement on the reconstruction based on the cost of saline implants?

- Will they pay for a prophylactic mastectomy of the non-cancerous breast without first having genetic screening (which takes over a month)?

- How difficult will it be to prevail upon your insurance company to allow your wife to stay in the hospital an extra night or two if she isn't ready to go home after surgery?

- What alternative treatments are available to your wife through the hospital and are they covered? (Cathy took acupuncture through MSKCC that was helpful for pain management, but we later learned that our insurance company doesn't reimburse for this.)

- Does your insurance company pay for the purchase of wigs? If so, is there a cap, and do the wigs need to be 100 percent synthetic, or can they be a combination of synthetic and real hair?

Once you get a handle on these "gross costs," you should be able to ballpark your net costs. Both the hospital and your insurance company will be able to walk you through these costs so that you can have a relatively accurate sense as to how much money you will be out. You may not like the initial answer, but you should have some basic knowledge in advance as to what financial impediments lay ahead. My experience is that your insurance company will push you toward a hospital that works for them… not necessarily one that you and your wife determine works best for you.

I am acutely aware how lucky we are that we have insurance and the financial wherewithal to afford this horrible disease. The notion of having your net worth depleted, or going into debt to pay for life-saving treatments, is depressing and seems so unfair, which reinforces the need to draft a financial emergency plan. And if your spouse isn't sick or diagnosed and is still working, buy disability insurance for her. You will need to buy it while she is still working because if she later quits her job to stay at home to raise children, you can maintain her disability insurance. Unfortunately, I never thought about this before Cathy got sick, nor did I have a formalized emergency plan.

Additionally, even if your wife doesn't have cancer, you should still have some life insurance on her life as well as your own. If your wife dies, you will have to replace her work in the home with hired help, and you will likely suffer professionally. I know that I took some solace in the fact that I had a life insurance policy for Cathy before she got sick, because I knew that I could rebound from the financial depletion of her illness over time if she lived, and would be paid by insurance if she didn't.

I also know that in ten or twenty years, I am not going to look back on this ordeal and even remotely think about our finances. However, I am going to look back and think about how I guided my wife and kids through a trying time. By enveloping them with love and optimism, I will view my role as husband and father as being successful. I know that I will recoup my lost earnings and be better in business because I will have gained an important perspective on life outside, which will allow me to disconnect from many of the day-to-day work-related pressures that can be corrosive to effective performance. While our society has inculcated all of us with a drive to make money and, in fact, to value wealth, true wealth is having your wife healthy and your family secure. I've come to realize that it's all in your perspective. I hope I can maintain this perspective for the rest of my life.

CHAPTER 9
FAITH AND FREINDSHIP

Cathy's dearest friend Caryl Orlando felt absolutely helpless when she found out that Cathy had cancer. Adding to Caryl's frustration was the fact that she just moved from Manhattan to Scarsdale and couldn't be here every day during treatment for her best friend. While Caryl had some knowledge about breast cancer, she saw how I was quarterbacking Cathy's treatment decisions and was confident that we were undertaking the right medical decisions. She wanted nothing more than to help Cathy, and to her great credit came up with a most remarkable way. She arranged for a "reading" from Chaim Yosef, a revered Kabbalah scholar of Yemenite origin from Brooklyn. Caryl told us that Chaim might be able to predict the outcome of Cathy's cancer, give us insight into our lives in a penetrating way, and would bless our home in a mystical way that would harness our positive energy. It sounded like a combination of fortune-telling and Jewish Feng Shui.

Cathy and I (me, especially) were more than a bit skeptical at first, as we had spent the previous three weeks since her diagnosis immersed in medical and statistical stuff. Our focus up until that point was on the real world, not the spiritual. We had done a fair amount of homework about surgery and were positive that we chose the right surgeons at the right hospital to perform the right surgery at the most opportune time. Cathy's fate was really out of our hands and we knew it. We also knew that the surgical outcome wasn't completely in the surgeon's hands either, as the true nature of Cathy's cancer wouldn't be known until well after surgery, when the pathology results came back.

We were within a few days of Cathy's surgery and the beginning of what promised to be a long and unpleasant journey with an uncertain outcome. In fact, there was so much uncertainty in our lives that I found myself grasping for answers and reassurance. I couldn't get either from doctors, friends, family or books. The only absolute point of certainty I could find was from God. I knew that I needed help here, so I prayed and drew a degree of comfort that I was turning our problems over to God after I had done all that I could do to the best of my abilities. I asked Him for a good outcome, and if that wasn't in His plan, I asked to let me be strong enough to provide strength and comfort to Cathy and my boys.

According to Caryl, Chaim represented an opportunity to look into the future and perhaps, see what God had in store for us. At a minimum, he would bless our home so as to ward off evil. Notwithstanding my skepticism, I really couldn't argue and win because Caryl had already convinced Cathy that Chaim could help us. I accepted that there was nothing that I could do... Chaim was coming!

Two days before Cathy's surgery, on a quiet, snowy night in Manhattan, Chaim arrived at our home, sat with us around our dining room table and spoke through his interpreter, Channie. Channie explained that Chaim only spoke Hebrew (and Arabic), and was legendary in both Brooklyn and Israel.

Chaim spoke for about ten minutes, then started our reading by asking me to open his Kabbalah, which is a collection of mystical teachings of rabbinical origin, based on esoteric interpretation of the Hebrew scriptures. I opened to a page at random and Chaim immediately said (through Channie) that he saw only two children in our home but knew that I had another son. He also said that the page I had chosen showed with clarity that my oldest son was in the Air Force. While a little impressed that he knew I had an older son, I plaintively told Chaim that my oldest son was not in the Air Force. He emphatically told me again that my son must be in the Air Force…but did allow that perhaps he flew helicopters instead of jets! Rather than argue with Chaim (which certainly have lead to an argument with Cathy), I softly said that he might not be right because my son Or is a counter-terrorist commando in the Israeli Army, not a pilot, but that I would ask Or if he had any thoughts of trying to switch into the Air Force (even though I knew that he didn't). Chaim wasn't upset so much as a bit confused—the numerology of the Kabbalah as per the random page I chose had told him that my son was a flyer. In hindsight, at that moment, I am certain Chaim believed the Kabbalah more than he believed me.

Chaim then went on to tell me things about my life, my mother, Brandon and Ryan, as well as things about my marriage and my past that were uncannily accurate. Except for his initial mistake about my son's vocation, he started to make me into a believer, or at least much less skeptical. For thirty minutes, he told me things about my past and present thoughts that I hadn't shared with anyone. Every time he changed topics, he asked me to open to a different page in his Kabbalah. This was extraordinary in several ways, not the least of which was that he was ignoring Cathy completely. He was sitting at our dining room table to read her future and instead was telling us about mine. He also spoke about Or and Brandon's futures in very reassuring ways, predicting that Or would recover from his leg injury (which Chaim accurately told me about with no prompting) and be able to rejoin his unit in "the Air Force," and that Brandon would overcome his learning disabilities and exceed our wildest expectations for success and happiness. I don't recall him making any predictions about Ryan, who at this point was fast asleep in his room.

His insight into my life and his predictions were great, but he offered nothing about Cathy, which actually concerned me; I was afraid he was concealing an unpleasant view of her future. So, I asked him point-blank,

"Is Cathy going to be all right?" At that point, all we had told him about Cathy is that she recently received a cancer diagnosis. He looked at her with penetrating brown eyes and asked her to open the Kabbalah. He studied the page she chose and said that "the mountains will fall," but in the aftermath, she would survive and make a complete recovery before the end of the year (this meant September, a full nine months away, because he was referring to the Jewish New Year.) He also told us definitively that Cathy's cancer would not spread.

Because Chaim's prognostications for Cathy, Or and Brandon had happy answers, and because I was yearning for reassurance, I believed that Chaim had accurate insight into the future. The only damper on my confidence in him was his "mistake" relative to Or serving in the Air Force. He wasn't a flyer and I knew he didn't want to be! I asked Chaim how he came up with this and why he was so positive about it. He reopened his Kabbalah to the first page I had picked that night, then explained to me that the numerology of the page addressed clearly that my son was a warrior from the sky. He repeated that it cannot be any other way, and showed me the page and pointed to certain words (which I didn't understand because they were in Hebrew). As he grew passionate and started arguing in Hebrew with Channie, I sat there quietly thinking about Or. Then, my mouth suddenly dropped open, as I realized that Or's unit is a Sayeret or commando unit, which is part of the larger branch of the army called the Sonchanim or paratroopers. And paratroopers really are "warriors from the sky." When I explained this to Chaim he gave a Channie a classic "never question me again while I'm working" look!

I went to bed that night concerned but confident in Chaim's vision that God would take care of Cathy and that she would be OK. While there was nothing scientific about it, Cathy and I drew a degree of comfort from Chaim's visit. If this was some sort of hoax, it was OK, because the power of positive thinking didn't hurt us one bit.

I feel that it's important to talk about this because as a husband and father going through a time of illness and uncertainty, everyone looked to me for guidance and reassurance. My family and friends would ask, "Is she going to be all right?" And I, like all men in a similar position, wanted to be able to make everything all right. My kids needed answers and reassurance, as did Cathy's parents, brother and friends. I wanted to be able to offer an encouraging report on an outcome that was far beyond my control; I wanted to take definitive steps to come as close as I could to controlling that outcome even after I was certain that I had exhausted all means available to me.

It was during this point that my relationship with God was most intense because I had nowhere else to turn, and I needed to pour my heart out and ask for things that were beyond anyone's control. My unstructured prayers were very comforting because they helped me format my thinking into discreet areas of concern. As I would pray for Cathy's health, I thought over and over about the medical choices we were making. As I prayed for my children's emotional welfare, I also thought constantly about how I spoke to them, what information to give them and when to give it. This quiet private time of reflection took on a positive pattern because I wouldn't ask God for things unless I had first taken responsible steps to achieve them. For example, I asked God to give me the strength to lead Cathy and the boys through this ordeal, and not to let me buckle under my new situational pressure and stress. But first I made sure that I was getting sufficient sleep, daily exercise, and watching my diet carefully. I knew that long periods of stress would wear down my immune system, so I took the steps within my control to bolster it.

Stress has a way of stripping away much of our defensive armor and readily exposes our flaws. The wear and tear of the stress of Cathy's illness threatened to take two negative aspects of my personality that I generally kept in check—being a control freak and a bit of an obsessive compulsive—and allow them to surface, perhaps even run rampant. At first I tried to convince myself that I had the ability to guide Cathy to a cure by getting her the best medical care possible and by making the smartest and "right" decisions. But pretty quickly after her diagnosis, I came to the crashing realization that this thing was much bigger than anything I'd ever dealt with and that, regardless of having the best medical care, Cathy might die and I couldn't stop it from happening. It suddenly became clear that if I were going to be part of Cathy's solution rather than another one of her problems, I needed to get my emotional house in order, because she couldn't waste any of her emotional energy worrying about and caring for me. Counseling, exercise and research were tools that I used to do this… but they weren't quite enough.

During the darkest months of Cathy's illness, I found myself obsessing about all kinds of little things because I couldn't control the biggest thing going on in our lives. With my world out of control and Brandon and Ryan looking constantly to me for reassurance, I struggled to find the right way to comfort them. At the suggestion of my friend Rabbi David Laine, while putting Brandon to sleep I prayed a prayer of thanksgiving to God, expressing gratitude for the many good things that we had in our lives. In fact, I specified many of those things, then humbly asked God to watch over all of us and to especially take care of Mommy. Brandon took great comfort in this and said "Amen" when I finished. The next night Ryan prayed with us, and a new nightly ritual was started. I drew reassurance from God, but more importantly, so did my boys. I would continue to pray even after they were asleep, and I know this helped me help Cathy… maybe it even resulted in her cure. Chaim, of course, would be certain of it!

CHAPTER 10

HELPFUL COMMENTS PEOPLE SAY

When speaking to a person who is dealing with cancer, some people feel compelled to say something about the disease when silence or a warm smile would be more appropriate. I noticed this over and over when Cathy got sick. In general, I think that people are good and want to make you feel better or alleviate your stress when they see you are in emotional pain. Unfortunately, with some people, their desire to ease your suffering can be mixed with a narcissistic need to demonstrate how much they "know" about cancer.

I found that when people in my life heard about Cathy's illness they reacted differently—some wonderfully, and some not. The good reactions were the most simple. Statements like, "I'm so sorry to hear that. You will be in my prayers and most hopeful thoughts," or, "You are lucky to have each other and to be so resourceful while you face this challenge," actually made me feel better; these expressions of support were upbeat and sensitive without prying into our need for a modicum of privacy. These expressions also didn't require me to respond, which was much appreciated.

Cathy and I decided that less is generally more when it came to interactions with friends immediately after finding out about her diagnosis. I'm convinced that simple, elegant support is all anyone really wants. Statements like "If there is anything I can do," are generally as disingenuous as they are ridiculous, because most people aren't accustomed to asking for help, and people who quickly make such blanket general offers to help don't understand the consequences of making them. Before asking if there is anything that they can do' a person would be well advised to consider how they would react if the answer came back, "Actually, I need a little help. Would you mind picking up Brandon from the therapist's office on Tuesday at 4:00 P.M. and taking him to gymnastics, then waiting with him until about 6:45 when I get there? I have a really important presentation at work, and Cathy can't get out of bed because it will be Day 2 after chemo." If the answer to that request would be "I'd love to, but I need to be at work myself," or "I have to pick up my own daughter from ballet lessons at that time," then the person offering help has rejected and humiliated the person they thought they were helping with their offer.

I was really disappointed with a former colleague at work, whom I had regarded as a friend. Michael called me when he heard that Cathy was sick in January and said, "If there is anything I can do for you and the kids, please let me know." I didn't ask him for anything because, like most people, I am unaccustomed to asking for help, and I wasn't completely sure what help I needed. He called again in April and suggested that we make plans to come visit him and his kids in New Jersey that summer, to enjoy his pool and "get out of the city." I asked him if his pool was heated and he told me it was and described how his daughters had him keep the pool really warm. I asked because I was thinking about a swim in May, when it is still sometimes cool outside. Since this was a second offer and it seemed sincere (even though I felt a bit like a poster boy for the Fresh Air Fund), and I was really in need of some diversions for my boys, I decided to take him up on his offer. I asked him if the boys and I could come over for a swim during the second weekend in May, as Cathy would be recovering from her last chemotherapy session.

His answer floored me and still causes me pain when I think about it. He said that he wouldn't be opening his pool for the season until the third weekend in May, since there were inchworms that fall from the trees in his yard in early May and he would have to skim his pool nightly for a week if he opened it any earlier to "accommodate" us. I didn't know how to respond, so I meekly said, "OK." I was so drained at that point from being a supportive husband and an entertaining, loving father, and I thought that my "friend" understood this. Perhaps he did, but he wasn't moved enough to open his pool early and skim a few inchworms! I asked so little of people during this crisis precisely because I didn't want the hurt of having anyone reject me. In hindsight, my friend's offer felt insincere, and I now interpret it this way; "Mark, in order to make me feel better about not being in your shoes, I am prepared to offer you and your kids a diversion, provided it comes at no cost and no inconvenience to me whatsoever."

During the months following Cathy's diagnosis, I spent much time trying not to be bitter and to be more understanding of people and their shortcomings. Initially after receiving and digesting her diagnosis, I felt and radiated bitterness because I felt that we had been singled out so unfairly. Looking back now, I know we were singled out, but were singled out with good fortune because although Cathy got cancer, we had the wherewithal to deal with it and have a very high probability that we beat it forever. At least in the beginning, however, the "Why Cathy?" part of all this probably contributed to my opening bouts with bitterness. My feelings were often amplified by the many inadvertently unkind or even silly comments that I heard from people both intimately and distantly involved in our lives.

During the rough parts of this experience, I made mental notes of all the ridiculous things people said to me in the hope of providing myself with some level of comfort. As discussed, not everyone thinks before they speak, and they cannot resist the temptation to draw a parallel of your experiences to their own, however irrelevant those experiences may be. Others feel that the way to make you feel better is to point out that there are people they know who have it much *worse* than you. I was exposed to more silly comments than I imagined possible, and started collecting some of the real jewels by writing them down in a notebook. When I was bitter, they weren't so funny, but as my bitterness abated after a few months, I was able to find humor in almost all of these comments:

Bradley (a work colleague at my company's Christmas party that Cathy insisted I attend, even though she had only been diagnosed five days earlier): Mark, Sharon told me what you are going through…I understand. I lost my wife to cancer.

Me: I'm sorry for your loss. Thanks for sharing.

—December 17, 2002

Me (while walking on Lexington Avenue two days after Cathy's surgery): Hi Lori, I got your message last night. Thanks for asking, but it wouldn't be a good idea to visit Cathy in the hospital, as she is really uncomfortable now.

Lori (a woman who knows Cathy socially but could be characterized as a friend of a friend at best): She's still in the hospital?

Me: Yes.

Lori: Have you been to visit her?

Me: Yes, I've been to visit my wife after major surgery for a potentially fatal disease.

Lori: I didn't mean it like that. I just meant that it is important for you to really be there for her.

Me: I agree. Thanks for sharing.   —January 10, 2003

Helpful Comments People Say

Ross (a midlevel executive at my company who works in Contract Administration): How are things at home?

Me: OK. This is a tough week. We start chemo tomorrow.

Ross: I know how tough that is. In 1992, my girlfriend died in my arms during the middle of her chemotherapy. But we never gave up hope.

Me: Thanks for sharing.

—February 4, 2003

James (a colleague at work): How's your wife? I heard what's going on.

Me: OK, James, thanks for asking. We are in the middle of chemotherapy and it is pretty rough but our resolve is strong.

James: I know exactly what you are going through.

Me (thinking that perhaps his wife had gone through this ordeal): Oh?

James: My cousin is in bad shape. He was doing really well after he went through chemo. Then a tumor the size of a golf ball popped up out of nowhere by his spine. He's paralyzed now, in agony, basically praying for death. Poor guy… he has young kids, too.

Me: I'm sorry for your cousin. Thanks for sharing.

—March 27, 2003

Carol (the executive secretary to a client; she lives in my neighborhood and had heard from her boss that Cathy was sick): Hi, Mark, how is your wife?

Me: Not bad, Carol, thanks for asking.

Carol: How are her spirits?

Me: She's a bit down now. We are in the middle of chemotherapy and it's a long process.

Carol: Did she lose her hair?

Me: Yes, she lost her hair at the beginning of chemo.

Carol: All of it?

Me: Yes.

Carol: I know what you can do to pick up her spirits... buy her some nice scarves. If that doesn't work... buy her a wig!

Me: Those are good ideas. Thanks for sharing.

—March 28, 2003

Linda (the parent of one of Brandon's schoolmates from first grade): Mark, I just heard about Cathy, I'm so sorry. How is she?

Me: She got through her surgery fine and we are in the midst of chemo, which is manageable, but rough.

Linda: I know how that can be. My aunt, she's sixty-six, just went through the same thing. She had a lumpectomy; thank God they got it on time. Did Cathy?

Me: Did Cathy what?

Helpful Comments People Say

Linda: Did she get the cancer before it spread?

Me: I hope so.
Linda: Did it spread to her lymph nodes?

Me: I'm uncomfortable discussing such personal medical topics. I hope you understand.

Linda: I understand. It's just that my aunt detected a lump while it was really small and had it taken care of right away. We all encouraged her to deal with it right away.

Me: That was good advice. You sound like a supportive niece. Thanks for sharing.

—April 7, 2003

Vinny (At Marinaro's Jewelers where I was having Cathy's watch serviced): How long have you had this watch now?

Me: About a year.

Vinny: Did your wife like it?

Me: Yes, very much. I actually bought it from you a week before I found out that she had breast cancer.

Vinny: Oh my god… did she die?

Me: No, Vinny, but she had a really tough year with surgery and chemotherapy. She is fine now.

Vinny: This damn cancer… it kills so many people. My sister's best friend just died of it.

Me: Died of what?

Vinny: Multiple Sclerosis.

Me: Vinny, that's not cancer.

Vinny: I know, but they should just find a goddam cure.

Me: I agree. I'm sorry about your friend's sister. Thanks for sharing.
—March 30, 2004

As I walked out of the store, I smiled because I knew that Vinny had just "made my book!"

I don't think that any of the people who said these things ever had bad intentions; rather, I think they were either never taught to think before speaking, or they get so nervous in a difficult situation that they just panic. There is also a chance that they are simply clueless. And because I saw no evil in any of the people who made unwittingly insensitive comments, I never really got angry with them. Of course, if I ever overheard anyone say a foolish thing to Cathy, that would have angered me. Cathy sensed this and was really careful not to share any of the idiotic comments that I'm sure she must have received.

My advice to men who are going through what I lived through is to find humor in these uncomfortable situations, and to realize that people are basically good and really don't mean any harm. A lifetime of boorishness, narcissism, or stupidity isn't likely to be masked when they are confronted with a delicate issue. The flip side of this is that you learn how to speak to someone who is undergoing a similar ordeal, and understand how to express support without being pedantic or asking questions that the respondent isn't comfortable answering.

During spring vacation, Cathy wasn't able to travel, so I took the boys for a mini-break to Florida while Cathy's wonderful, devoted friend Kim came to New York from Los Angeles to stay with her. While in Florida, I met the head tennis pro, Mario, at my father's country club, The Polo Club (even though they don't play any polo there whatsoever). We struck up a conversation because years earlier Mario was the head tennis pro of Aspatuck Tennis Club in Westhampton Beach, where I was Club President. Mario was the pro there before I joined, and is universally revered by many of the old time members. During our conversation, Mario asked me if my wife came down to Florida with me. I told him that she hadn't because she hadn't been sick. He surprised me by asking, "How sick?" And when I replied, "Very sick, she has breast cancer," he told me about his wife, who succumbed to ovarian cancer ten years earlier. We then spoke about the strains of parenting children and supporting a wife during tough times. He was so gentle and open in a completely sensitive way that I cannot remember ever making such a quick but certain connection with another man. He had walked the walk I was walking, and did it as well as he could. Unfortunately for him, his journey ended badly.

I remember thinking that only those who have shared similar experiences can have the credibility to have a meaningful conversation about what you are going through. That isn't to say that someone who has never lived through the illness of a spouse can't listen caringly to you, but the experiences of supporting a loved one through a health crisis is so unique that one ought to be careful in trying to demonstrate empathy when it isn't grounded in experience.

CHAPTER 11

LIFE AFTER CANCER
AND A PAINFUL LOOK IN THE MIRROR

On January 31, 2004, just over a year after Cathy's surgery and almost four-teen months since our ordeal with her breast cancer began, Cathy had an experience while walking our dog Sami in Carl Shultz Park, near our apartment. She described it to me as we sat quietly that evening in our living room.

In the park, Cathy met and struck up a conversation with a forty-four-year-old woman who had two dogs. Perhaps this woman sensed that Cathy was a breast cancer survivor from her very short hair, because while her dogs and Sami were romping in the dog run, she shared with Cathy the fact that she underwent bilateral mastectomies at MSKCC seven years earlier. She had also undergone a rigorous course of chemotherapy followed by aromotase inhibitors, which suppress the body's manufacture of androgen, which gets converted into estrogen (tumors flourish in an estrogen-rich environment). She explained that her cancer returned by attacking her lungs three years after her initial bout with breast cancer. She fought the return of the cancer with another brutal round of chemotherapy, which again took her hair and vitality, but she got "through it."

The woman went on to add that a recent bone scan detected that the cancer had returned yet again and attacked her bones, which, when taken with the lung metastasis, does not bode well for her long-term survival. I was surprised that in a relatively short conversation, this woman shared such personal details with my wife, and that once she learned that Cathy underwent bilateral mastectomies and chemotherapy only a year ago, she still felt compelled to continue with her very personal tale of plight.

As Cathy told me this unsettling story, I couldn't help but feel badly about the way I sometimes treat her. This was a stark reminder that her cancer could come back really at any time. I began thinking about how I'm often too hard on Cathy for insignificant oversights like misplacing articles of clothing while putting away the laundry, or other little annoyances like leaving papers out on the kitchen counter and obscuring my "things." Sometimes I would also take out my business frustrations on her, and use the way she organized our house as a target for my anger. The notion that Cathy's remaining lifespan might be less than ten years is horrible enough, but to think that I actually caused her stress over trivial matters during what may be a relatively short life is actually pathetic. Intellectually, I know that the location of my socks, mail and cell phone don't mean anything, but I had to teach myself to stop obsessing about inconsequential things, and this was a difficult pattern for me to break. I was able to realize that controlling the little things gave me a greater sense of control over my life. And interestingly, while Cathy was sick, I didn't put any pressure on her relative to taking care of me, but once I felt she was out of the woods physically, I again began expecting her to play the role in our household exactly as she had played it before she got sick.

Cathy's cancer was supposed to forever change my outlook on life, shifting my focus only to important and meaningful things. I was supposed to learn from the year of constant fear that my wife might die, take a larger view of life and become a kinder, more compassionate husband. And I would actually be that type of person for weeks at a time, until I would ultimately "fall off the wagon." Suddenly, in the second year after Cathy's cancer diagnosis, I felt a tremendous incongruity between her new reality and refined focus on life and my propensity to revert to our life pre-cancer. Intellectually and emotionally, I knew that I could never go back to that life—I wasn't even certain that it was something I wanted to do—yet

I felt a pull towards familiarity and "normalcy" after living through a year of consistent turmoil.

I recognized that Cathy's outlook on life had changed for the better; she was determined to move forward with vigor and savor every minute of every day. But I resisted, or at least didn't go along with her vigorous change of priorities, by blunting it with immature and sometimes counter-productive behavior. Ironically, I had always regarded myself as being more adaptive than Cathy and more accepting of change than she, yet it was Cathy who had changed decisively and now saw the world with more clarity than I had. My displeasure with my pettiness and my sincere desire to change—to move on like Cathy did—drove me to examine closely the issues that were driving my behavior. Once I understood the issues, it was relatively easy to draw a conclusion and, in some instances, make a resolution to aid myself in moving past these emotionally blocking problems. I actually wrote it all down to aid myself in going forward:

- **Issue:** I am under pressure because I have lost so much ground at work; last year was a bad year. **Conclusion:** Actually, last year (2003) worked out well financially, given the fragile state of the economy and the few months when I functioned really poorly. **Resolution:** I will take a five-year view, relative to the economics of cancer, and shouldn't remotely care that I am slightly behind the lofty expectations that I had before Cathy got sick.
- **Issue:** I am drained from having held together our family during 2003. **Conclusion:** Actually, notwithstanding Cathy's illness, she did a terrific job of holding things together and did as much as she physically could. It was by no means all me. In fact, the stress I was under paled in comparison to Cathy's stress during the past year. **Resolution:** I will try not to put any further stress on her.
- **Issue:** For a year, all of the focus was on Cathy and our kids with none on me. **Conclusion:** How pathetic that, at forty-one years old, I needed attention and recognition for having to do what any decent man would

have to do at a time of crisis. **Resolution:** I will stop thinking and acting like a child.

● **Issue:** My goals and needs were either derailed or delayed while Cathy was undergoing treatment. **Conclusion:** When we got married, I don't remember anyone promising that marriage and family would always be easy, and would accommodate all of my other goals and needs all of the time. **Resolution:** I will realistically adjust my goals and needs.

Seeing these issues in black and white showed me that I had to learn to accept that Cathy's post-cancer reality is also my reality, and that every time she feels an ache or a pain, it causes her tremendous anxiety. She lives with the fear that her cancer could return any time, and so do I. Upon hearing of Cathy's illness, one of my former bosses at work, Anthony Saytanides, compared our post-cancer anxiety to how a person feels after they've been mugged: "They are forever looking over their shoulder." While I felt mugged by having had my wife get sick, I knew that Cathy's sense of insecurity must be much more profound.

The post-cancer anxiety affects your reaction to all health-related issues and concerns. Typically, we ignore aches and pains and are conditioned to write them off as "nothing." When we were children, the pains in our legs were said to be "growing pains." As we grow older, we ascribe many of our maladies to pollen, soreness, being overtired, stressed, or just having aches from the flu. But after someone in your family suddenly goes from being asymptomatic and perfectly healthy to being diagnosed with cancer, you develop a heightened sense of paranoia that extends not only to your spouse and yourself, but also to your children. When your four-year-old has a headache, you find yourself with a nervous stomach, wondering if he or she has a brain tumor.

While a part of me thinks that this heightened sense of self-awareness and fear is only going to be short-lived, I know better. I asked my mother if she still panics every time she has a new ache or pain, and she immediately answered, "Yes." She had cancer in 1969 and still has a heightened sensitivity to anything that might be wrong with her. She added that she has "learned how to deal with it a little bit better each year." This makes sense to me, as I've learned that people learn how to deal with just about everything that is thrown at them. The human spirit is remarkably adaptive.

Addiction

Cathy had much postoperative pain from her mastectomies, which included blinding headaches accompanying her chemotherapy, as well as significant physical pain after her reconstruction and oophorectomy. Once she left the hospital after her initial surgery, she found the only painkiller that really worked for her was Dilaudid, an opiate that she took in pill form. It increased her pain threshold and completely altered Cathy's perception of pain, making her feel pretty good when she otherwise would have been in a low-grade state of misery. In addition, it soothed the blistering headaches that she got during chemo.

While we understood Dilaudid's efficacy, we also understood that because it is opium based, it is highly addictive. Cathy voiced concern about this from the very beginning, but was basically glad-handed by everyone in MSKCC with comments like, "Our first concern is treating your cancer; we'll take care of any related problems like addiction later." MSKCC's major concern was to rid her body of cancer with addiction to anything coming in a distant second. Therefore, because our respected team of physicians didn't seem overly concerned with the potential for addiction, I pretty much put the possibility of it out of my mind, which was a mistake. It meant that Cathy, if susceptible to addiction (which she was) would be the only one to monitor her downward spiral into it. My naiveté was never more obvious because the last one to admit to addiction is an addict. Looking back, I realize I had left the fox to guard the henhouse.

Add to these issues the fact that modern medicine is totally fragmented, and what you have is a recipe for disaster. Any enterprising, newly addicted patient could easily play several physicians and pharmacists off each other in order to get virtually unlimited prescriptions to painkillers. When a pretty woman and mother of two, living on the Upper East Side of Manhattan, has been dealt a cancer diagnosis before forty years old and asks a doctor for some pain relief, the doctor generally complies with the assumption that she is a responsible person who can self-regulate.

In September, after "the transfer" and oophorectomy, Cathy, who had previously been taking 4 milligrams of Dilaudid a day in 2-milligram pills, was sent home with 4-milligram pills instead. This mistake seemed innocent enough. Perhaps it was the anxiety of being home and not feeling 100 percent, but she took two 4-milligram pills, which not only worked fine for the pain, but produced an almost instant euphoric effect associated with opiates, which of course was the beginning of her addiction. By Thanksgiving, she was surreptitiously up to 12 milligrams a day... and 16 by Christmas. She had her surgeon, plastic surgeon, oncologist, and general physician all pretty much fooled into thinking they were the only ones prescribing pain meds for her. Finally, they all started to catch on and, instead of confronting her, just stopped prescribing.

At that point, facing our Christmas vacation, Cathy realized that she couldn't go away without any Dilaudid because she was completely addicted and didn't want to have withdrawal seizures while we were in Hawaii. With me totally oblivious to her addiction—largely because I was in my own world trying to get back on track with business—Cathy went to a psychopharmacologist to help wean her.

In early January, after we got back from our trip, Cathy tearfully admitted to me that she was addicted, but was getting professional help to deal with it. Before her admission of addiction, a tension had developed in our marriage, and I am still not certain why. Was it because she was preoccupied with her addiction or craving for more drugs? Was it because I went into a tizzy of self-absorbed behavior, or was it because many of the problems we had with our marriage before Cathy got sick were put on a backburner for a year and allowed to simmer? I don't know the answer to these questions, but I suspect that her addiction played a role in the buildup of tension between us. I was never really upset with her for not telling me sooner; she knew, that if I knew I would have made certain that she undertake steps to deal with her addiction right away. Drug addicts only try to break their addiction when they have no other choice, and Cathy's choices ran out only when she couldn't readily replenish her supply of Dilaudid.

Cathy's drug dependency and its numbing effects, combined with her new perspective on life and my reluctance to embrace that, produced significant marital stress. Between menopause, drug addiction and my preoccupation with regaining traction in my career, communication and intimacy was not among the top of our priorities. Somehow, in the autumn of 2004, all of these elements that had been simmering started to boil over all at once. The major pressures were off and I had only to deal with lots of smaller pressures, but I didn't have much energy left to tackle them. I knew that I needed help because I felt that the glue holding me together emotionally during a year of turmoil, had suddenly stopped working.

When the problem was definable like "Cathy has cancer and needs surgery," I was able to stand and fight. Now I was having trouble facing pressures and problems that were almost ordinary in scope, as I felt that I had nowhere to turn except within myself. I felt like I had been driving for hours on the interstate at ninety miles per hour, and was now being forced to drive fifty-five. And while fifty-five is an acceptable pace, it seemed like

I was going backwards.

I went to a new psychiatrist for counseling because I wanted a fresh perspective from someone who didn't know me. I wanted someone who could bluntly explain why I was behaving the way I was, when I knew that I should have been responding as a gentle and caring husband whose prayers had been answered. After all, my wife—my kids' mother—had survived breast cancer.

Brandon was still seeing his psychologist, Cathy was seeing her psychiatrist and a psychopharmacologist for her drug addiction, and now I was back in therapy as well. The amount of money I was spending on counseling was staggering, but I needed to make certain that Brandon had an outlet for his emotions, that Cathy stayed sane and drug-free, and that I could function and be happy. Psychiatric treatment for stress is important, but spending a boatload of money each week on counseling brings its own stresses. I joked to my father that I wanted to take my family to Europe for a few weeks so that I could save money!

People generally regard going from a steady, predictable life into a high-stakes, unpredictable life as stressful. What I learned from having a wife who had lived through cancer and its treatments is that when your life slows from ninety miles per hour to fifty-five, it stays just as stressful because at slower speeds, the world doesn't feel quite right. You understand that you went through a horrible time, but you can't understand why you aren't able to seize each post-cancer moment and easily embrace it as being truly glorious.

I found that when you step away from the situation, you can finally acknowledge to yourself that it took time to accept that cancer is part of your wife's life and your own. So why shouldn't it take at least the same amount of time to regulate back into life after you've dealt with the onslaught of cancer's diagnosis and treatment? You try to get back to the perfect point in your marriage where love and understanding was the rule of the day, sex was perfect, and communication was open and effective, but you find great frustration in getting back to this point because you realize that this marriage "nirvana" didn't exist before your wife got sick.

Like most couples, Cathy and I had some problems that we were addressing prior to her illness, but because cancer was so prepossessing, we ignored those problems while I supported Cathy during her battle with the disease. We didn't acknowledge that the problems we had prior to her disease were being put on a backburner and might return. But since my basic nature is optimistic, I am certain that we can get through any and all distractions and difficulties, and view our lives together as a celebration.

Cancer clears certain obstacles to happiness in a marriage in that it lets you focus more intensely on the important things in your life. However, it also brings up issues that can't easily be ignored. The most pronounced difficulty is living with the knowledge that if cancer hadn't invaded our marriage, our life would be easier and far more pleasant. But I am now acutely aware that before Cathy was diagnosed with cancer, I didn't have the ability to see just how "pleasant" my life was, or how easy it should have been to derive happiness from my predictable days. This causes its own set of problems because it cries out that I shouldn't have needed a near catastrophe to see just how good our lives really were. It is a bit embarrassing to face up to this realization and it makes it awkward to talk to people about your life. You realize that others have it much worse and that when things were much better, you didn't even know it. I think I finally understand what people mean when they speak about "stopping to smell the roses."

Follow-Up Visits

Since all cancers are different, and oncologists and surgeons don't treat and see patients in a uniform manner, you can expect a range of time between follow-up visits. Cathy sees her oncologist every four months. When something isn't quite right, she orders a set of tests, which brings us back to the state of insecurity and helplessness that we tried so hard to forget. Reality has a way of interfering with denial.

Early detection is every bit as important in diagnosing a recurrence of cancer as it is in diagnosing cancer in the first place. In normal life, one doesn't panic or overreact to every little potential malady as if it were cancer. This is in stark contrast to being a post-operative and chemotherapy cancer survivor, where any symptom could mean the worst possible scenario and you are hypersensitive to everything. And since the odds of a recurrence are between 1 in 10 and 1 in 20, and that these recurrences often occur within the first five years after diagnosis and treatment, neither patient nor physician can ignore or brush off a symptom that might be consistent with a recurrence or a metastasis of breast cancer. What happens when a patient complains that she is fatigued and achy? The oncologist might ask where you are achy, or ask if you are achy around your thighs, sternum or shoulders. Since someone with the flu might be achy everywhere, the oncologist, owing to the high statistical possibility that there has been a recurrence of cancer, will have the patient come in for blood work, a body scan and a brain scan using magnetic resonance imaging.

These unpleasant procedures, which include drinking lots of barium sulfate to create contrast for scans are stressful, time consuming and expensive—so much so that the second time a patient feels rotten or achy, they might just wait a few days until they call their oncologist. Eventually, assuming there has been no recurrence, most patients adjust and become less fearful of any atypical feeling they might have. But the fear, as discussed earlier, never goes away completely.

Assuming there is no pain, a cancer patient, after treatments are over, will see their oncologist for follow-up visits at an interval that works for both patient and doctor. Cathy's oncologist is younger than Cathy, which is good because we expect and hope their relationship will be a long and caring one, marked by being uneventful. As cancer treatments become more effective and patients live longer, oncologists will likely become overwhelmed with treating new patients and seeing those who have survived the initial treatments after cancer. I expect that within the next ten years, a sub-specialty of oncology will develop, which will focus exclusively on patient monitoring. It will be the ultimate tribute to the researchers, physicians and patients who made successfully treating, curing and managing breast cancer a reality.

As I write this, I am fully cognizant that we are only at the beginning of understanding how to deal with our fear of recurrence. A recurrence, which can come in the form of either a local or distant metasis, generally means that the cancer is not curable and is a chronic condition that needs to be managed. With a distant metasis, which is often to the lungs, liver or bones, a patient is immediately reclassified as having Stage IV cancer. In Stage IV, the survival statistics drop off considerably.

Accordingly, Cathy will have blue days, and so will I. I'm resolved to being understanding and sympathetic to her blue moods, and to constantly trying to be the sort of loving husband that she deserves. Her cancer has given me a perspective of which I sometimes lose sight… but not for long. Cathy's illness will ultimately make me a better husband—so much so that in forty years, I might be able to look back and see how this horrible disease has added a dimension and richness to our lives that can only be achieved through overcoming adversity… together.